SENSORY TESTING METHODS: SECOND EDITION

Edgar Chambers IV and Mona Baker Wolf, Editors

ASTM Stock No.: MNL26

ASTM International
100 Barr Harbor Drive
PO Box C700
West Conshohocken, PA 19428-2959

Printed in the U.S.A.

Library of Congress Cataloging-in-Publication Data

Sensory testing methods/Edgar Chambers IV and Mona Baker Wolf,
    editors. — 2nd ed.
    (ASTM manual series; MNL 26)
    Rev. ed. of: Manual on sensory testing methods. 1968.
    "Sponsored by Committee E18 on Sensory Evaluation of Materials and
    Products."
    Includes bibliographical references and index.
    ISBN 0-8031-2068-0
    1. Senses and sensation—Testing.   2. Sensory evaluation.
    I. Chambers IV, Edgar.   II. Wolf, Mona Baker, 1949–   .   III. ASTM
    Committee E18 on Sensory Evaluation of Materials and Products.
    IV. Manual on sensory testing methods.   V. Series.
    BF233.M48   1996
    670'.28'7—dc20

                                                                        96-32386
                                                                        CIP

Printed in Philadelphia, PA
September 1996
Second Printing
Printed in Lancaster, PA
June 2005

Foreword

The second edition of the manual on *Sensory Testing Methods* has taken many years to complete. It is impossible to list all the individuals who had a part in its revision. In the period between the first edition of this book and this second edition a number of books have been written, research articles published, and conferences and workshops held. All of the authors, presenters, and participants ultimately contributed to the knowledge base for this book. The members past and present of ASTM Committee E18 on the Sensory Evaluation of Materials and Products all have contributed to the development of this manual although it certainly does not represent the views of every member.

Special mention must be given to Jackie Earhardt, formerly of General Mills, who started the revision of the manual. Also, the editors wish to thank Gene Groover and Jason Balzer who typed and retyped the many versions of this second revision.

Edgar Chambers IV, Kansas States University, and Mona Baker Wolf, WolfSensory, are the editors of this second edition.

Contents

Introduction	1
Chapter 1—General Requirements for Sensory Testing	3
Chapter 2—Forced Choice Discrimination Methods	25
Chapter 3—Scaling	38
Chapter 4—Threshold Methods	54
Chapter 5—Descriptive Analysis	58
Chapter 6—Affective Testing	73
Chapter 7—Statistical Procedures	79
Index	113

Introduction

Sensory evaluation, or sensory analysis as it often is called, is the study of human (and sometimes other animal) responses to products or services. It usually is used to answer one of three broad categories of questions related to products: "What is the product in terms of its perceived characteristics," "Is the product different from another product," and "How acceptable is the product (or is it preferred to some other product)." Those three broad questions are critical to the development, maintenance, and performance of most products.

Although much of the early science on which sensory evaluation is based was developed by psychologists using simple taste solutions, and much of the development of sensory methods has taken place by sensory scientists working in the food industry, the methods have been adapted to a number of other categories of products and services. Industries producing products and services as varied as personal care, paint, household cleaners, hospitality management, paper and fabrics, and air quality use sensory methods to provide information about their goods or services. In fact, any product or service that can be looked at, felt, smelled, tasted, heard, or any combination of those sensory modalities (that is, almost all products and services) can be analyzed using sensory methods.

The science of sensory evaluation consists of a broad spectrum of methods and techniques that encompass psychology; statistics; product sciences, such as, food science or cosmetic chemistry; other biological sciences; physics and engineering; ergonomics; sociology; and other mathematics, sciences, and humanities. Some of its most powerful methods require an understanding of how people use language and other communication.

This manual assumes the reader is interested in obtaining a general knowledge of sensory evaluation methods. It provides a base of practical techniques and the controls that are necessary to conduct simple sensory studies. For more advanced knowledge, other resources will be necessary.

For those interested in more knowledge than can be provided in this manual, the following list of books may be helpful. Also at the end of each chapter is a bibliography that also may be read for greater understanding. These lists are not intended to be complete listings of the literature available.

Bibliography

Amerine, M. A., Pangborn, R. M., and Roessler, E. B., *Principles of Sensory Evaluation of Food,* Academic Press, New York, 1965.

Hootman, R. C., *Manual on Descriptive Analysis Testing for Sensory Evaluation,* American Society for Testing and Materials, Philadelphia, 1992.

Jellinek, G., *Sensory Evaluation of Foods Theory and Practice,* Ellis Horwood Ltd., Deerfield Beach, FL, 1985.

Lawless, H. T. and Klein, B. P., *Sensory Science Theory and Applications in Foods,* Marcel Dekker, New York, 1991.

Lyon, D. H., Francombe, M. A., Hasdell, T. A., and Lawson, K., *Guidelines for Sensory Analysis in Food Product Development and Quality Control,* Chapman & Hall, London, 1992.

Meilgaard, M., Civille, G. V., and Carr, B. T., *Sensory Evaluation Techniques, 2nd ed.,* CRC Press, Boca Raton, FL, 1991.

Moskowitz, H. R., *Product Testing and Sensory Evaluation of Foods Marketing and R&D Approaches,* Food & Nutrition Press, Westport, CT, 1983.

Moskowitz, H. R. (ed.), *Applied Sensory Analysis of Foods,* Vols. I and II, CRC Press, Boca Raton, FL, 1988.

Munoz, A. M., Civille, G. V., and Carr, B. T., *Sensory Evaluation in Quality Control,* Van Nostrand Reinhold, New York, 1992.

Piggott, J. R., *Sensory Analysis of Foods, 2nd ed.,* Elsevier, New York, 1988.

Poste, L. M., Mackie, D. A., Butler, G., and Larmond, E., *Laboratory Methods for Sensory Analysis of Food,* Canada Communication Group-Publishing Centre, Ottawa, Canada, 1991.

Stone, H. and Sidel, J. L., *Sensory Evaluation Practices, 2nd ed.,* Academic Press, San Diego, CA, 1993.

Watts, B. M., Ylimaki, G. L., Jeffery, L. E., and Elias, L. G., *Basic Sensory Methods for Food Evaluation,* The International Research Centre, Ottawa, Canada, 1989.

Yantis, J. E. (ed.), *The Role of Sensory Analysis in Quality Control,* Manual 14, American Society for Testing and Materials, Philadelphia, 1992.

Chapter 1—General Requirements for Sensory Testing

PHYSICAL CONDITIONS

Sensory testing requires special controls of various kinds. If they are not employed, results may be biased or sensitivity may be reduced. Most of these controls depend on, or are affected by, the physical setting in which tests are conducted. The major environmental controls include elimination of irrelevant odor or light stimulation, elimination of psychological distraction, and providing a comfortable work environment.

This section describes, in general terms, the conditions that are desirable and indicates how they usually are attained in laboratories that have been designed especially for sensory testing. When sensory testing must be done using facilities not designed for that purpose, control is more difficult, but not necessarily impossible. In that situation, researchers should improvise to approximate the optimal conditions as closely as possible.

Location

Many factors need to be considered related to the location of the testing laboratory, because its location may determine how easy or difficult it is to establish and maintain respondents and physical controls. In addition, there are two general considerations: accessibility and freedom from confusion.

The laboratory should be located so that the majority of the available test respondents can reach it conveniently, with minimal disturbance in normal routines. Inconveniently located laboratories will reduce the respondent population substantially because individuals will not want to participate. In addition, motivation and performance of respondents may be adversely affected.

It usually is best to locate the laboratory where there is not a heavy flow of traffic in order to avoid confusion and noise. For example, laboratories within a company facility generally should not be placed next to a lobby or cafeteria, because of the possibility of disturbing the tests. However, this requirement may appear to conflict with accessibility. Laboratories may be near those areas for accessibility purposes without compromising testing conditions if special procedures to control noise and confusion, such as sound-proofing and waiting rooms, are used.

Laboratory Layout

One objective in designing a laboratory is to arrange the test area to achieve efficient physical operations. A second objective is to design the facility to avoid distraction of testers by the operation of the laboratory equipment/personnel or

3

by outside persons. A third objective is to minimize mutual distraction among respondents.

The testing area should be divided into at least two parts: one a work area for storage and sample preparation, and the other for actual testing. Those areas must be separated adequately to eliminate interference if preparation involves cooking, odorous, and visual materials.

For most types of tests, individual panel booths are essential to avoid mutual distraction among testers. However, they should not be built so that respondents feel completely isolated from others.

It is important to provide a space outside the testing room where test respondents can wait either before or after the test without disturbing those who are testing. This allows room for social interaction, payment of stipends, or other business that should not take place inside the actual room(s) used for testing.

Odor Control

For many types of product tests, the testing area must be kept as free from odors as possible. That sometimes is difficult to attain, and the degree to which the sensory professional may compromise with an ideal total lack of odor is a matter of judgment. Some desirable practices are given here, but many circumstances will require special solutions.

An air temperature and humidity control system with activated carbon filters is a means of odor control. A slight positive air pressure in the testing room to reduce inflow of air from the sample preparation room and other areas is recommended. Air from the sample preparation room should be vented to an area outside the testing facility and should not pass through the filters leading into the testing room. Intake air should not come from areas outside the building that are near high odor production areas such as manufacturing exhaust vents or garbage dumpsters.

All materials and equipment inside the room should either be odor-free or have a low odor level. If highly odorous products are to be examined, partitions to help control odor transmission are necessary. Those partitions may be coated with an odorless material that can be replaced if it becomes contaminated.

Air in the testing room may become contaminated from the experimental samples themselves, for example, when testing perfumes. Procedures must be developed that are suitable for the materials and the tests, so that odorous samples are exposed for a minimum time and the atmosphere of the room can be returned to normal before other samples are tested.

Lighting

Most testing does not require special lighting. The objective should be to have an adequate, even, comfortable level of illumination such as that provided by most good lighting systems.

Special light effects may be desired to emphasize or hide irrelevant differences in color and other aspects of appearance. Emphasis may be achieved with spotlighting, changes in spectral illumination (for example, changing from incandescent to fluorescent lighting or changing types of fluorescent bulbs), or changes in the position of the light source.

To reduce or hide differences one may simply use a very low level of illumination, special lights such as sodium lamps, or may adjust the color or illumination either with colored bulbs, or by attaching colored filters over standard lights. Changing the color of light may help reduce appearance differences caused by hue (for example, red or amber), but may do little to mask appearance differences related to appearance characteristics such as degree of brownness, uniformity of color (spotting), or geometric appearance characteristic such as surface cracking or conformation differences.

General Comfort

There must be an atmosphere of comfort and relaxation in the testing room that will encourage respondents to concentrate on the sensory tasks. A controlled temperature and humidity is desirable to provide consistent comfort. Care should be taken in selecting chairs and stools, designing work areas, and providing other amenities (coat closets, rest rooms, secure areas for personal belongings, etc.) to ensure that respondents feel comfortable and can concentrate only on testing.

Bibliography

Eggert, J. and Zook, K., *Physical Requirement Guidelines for Sensory Evaluation Laboratories,* *ASTM STP 913,* American Society for Testing and Materials, Philadelphia, 1986.
Larmond, E., "Physical Requirements for Sensory Testing," *Food Technology,* Vol. 27, No. 11, Nov. 1973, pp. 28–32.

TEST RESPONDENTS

Analytical Tests (Difference and Description)

Selection

Respondents in analytical tests must qualify for those tests by completing a series of tasks that help to predict testing capability. That process is called screening. Depending on the task, respondents must show an ability to discriminate among stimuli or to describe and quantify the characteristics of products. These methods require that a respondent deal analytically with complex stimuli; hence, any series of tasks using only simple stimuli can only partly determine a person's value as a respondent. It is necessary to take into consideration the many factors that may influence testing performance, and this can be done only by using representative tests on representative materials.

The selection process is started with a large group of people, the objective being to rank candidates in order of skill. The size of the initial screening group may affect the efficiency of the ultimate panel because the larger the number of candidates the greater the probability of finding respondents of superior testing ability. Do not excuse anyone from the screening tests on the grounds that he/she is automatically qualified because of special experience or position.

Re-qualification of panel members should be done periodically or, where possible, continually. Examination of each respondents' performance either in actual tests or in additional screening tests will indicate if the respondent needs additional training or instruction, or ultimately must be dismissed from the panel.

It must be remembered that the goal of screening usually is not to find candidates that are hypersensitive to various stimuli. Rather, screening is conducted to find candidates who are capable of conducting the test (for example, no allergies to the products, time to conduct the test, etc.), are able to discriminate among products and attributes, and for some tests, respondents who have sufficient verbal and analytical skills to describe and quantify those differences.

Discriminative Ability

One basic procedure for determining if respondents can discriminate among samples is the triangle test. The differences represented in the screening tests should be similar to those likely to be encountered in the actual operation of the panel. For example, if the panel is to be used for only one product, that product should be used to design screening tests. The tests should cover as broad a range of the anticipated differences as possible. For example, variation in ingredients, processing, storage or weathering conditions, or product age may be used.

Each test should represent a recognizable difference to enough respondents so that the "panel" as a whole will establish a significant difference. However, the percentage of correct responses should not be so high (for example, above 80%) that the difference was obvious to almost everyone. The test should be easy enough for some people to find differences, but difficult enough so that everyone does not find the differences.

Candidates are ranked on the basis of percentage of correct responses. Those people obtaining the highest percentage of correct responses are selected, with a provision that no one scoring less than some specified correct percentage (60% sometimes is used) would be used. It is recommended that each candidate take all, or nearly all, of the tests. Otherwise, the percentage correct may produce a biased basis of comparison, because tests are likely to vary in degree of difficulty. If product characteristics are such that sensory adaptation is not a problem, each person can do multiple tests in the same test session. It is recommended that selection be based on at least 20 to 24 tests per respondent.

A second procedure for screening has candidates describe or score characteristics of samples that represent a range of some specific descriptive characteristics. The rating scales used in the screening tests should be similar to those that will be used when the panel is finally operating. A series of four to six samples, all variations of a single product type and representing a range of levels of some characteristic, is made or selected. If the panel is to be used on more than one product type, this series of samples should be of the product type of major interest. Alternatively, the experiment should be repeated on two or three product types. Each candidate scores the series of samples for several simple pre-selected characteristics of the product.

The characteristics, or attributes, that are chosen must be ones that untrained respondents can understand. A minimum of four replications of scoring is recommended to enable further analysis of the data. The data for each candidate are subjected separately to analysis of variance. The level of significance for samples is used as the measure of the panel member skill.

Panel members also may be screened for their ability to describe characteristics of products. In the food and fragrance industries, a series of bottles containing odorous materials, some which are common and some which are less common, often is used for this screening. Potential respondents are asked to smell each bottle and name, describe, or associate the odor. Respondents are ranked according to their ability to characterize the odor materials, with preference being given to those candidates who can name or describe the odor rather than simply associate it with other products or odors. Similar series can be established for industries where appearance, sound, or tactile sensation are to be scored. Under no circumstances should respondents be selected who are unable to describe or associate most sensations. Those individuals may be unable, either physically or psychologically, to perform descriptive tasks well.

Number of Panel Members

Investigators use different criteria to determine panel size. There is no "magic" number. The number of panel members that are used varies considerably from one laboratory to another. Each situation may have its own particular needs. Also, panel size may depend on the number of qualified persons available. A panel should never include a person, or persons, with less than satisfactory qualifications just to achieve a predetermined panel size.

Basically, the number of respondents should depend on the variability of the product, the reproducibility of judgments, and whether there are basic differences between panel members. When a panel is first organized such information usually is unavailable, and panel size often is determined by the number of qualified persons available. Specific instructions regarding panel size are not appropriate because of the many factors that must be considered. For information purposes, descriptive tests typically have four or more respondents and often have eight to ten or more. Discrimination tests rarely use less than 20 to 25 respondents (and often up to 40 respondents) unless the products are shown to be different with fewer numbers.

If at all possible, a pool of qualified persons (depending on the amount of work anticipated and the number of people available) should be maintained. Individuals used for a given test or series of tests then are drawn in regular rotation.

This has obvious advantages, including the ready availability of replacements in emergencies (replacements should take the entire test if it is a series, not just one or a few parts), improved motivation through reduction of the test load on any one person, and the capability of handling peak loads of testing by conducting several simultaneous tests with different panels trained equivalently.

Affective Tests

Selection

Preference or acceptance testing requires different selection criteria than discrimination or descriptive tests. The criterion of respondent selection for studies of liking should be the representativeness of the panel to some consumer population and the elimination of respondents with allergies or illness that would preclude them from testing the material involved. The approaches used in selection for discrimination and descriptive tests are contrary to the objectives of preference or acceptance tests. Affective tests are used to determine direction of choice or the extent to which a product appeals to some population.

Definition of the population of interest is required, although many compromises are accepted in routine work. Sophisticated sampling procedures are available, but they are beyond the scope of this manual and often are not needed for initial guidance in research development or quality assurance testing. Often it becomes a matter of assuring random selection of respondents, working within the limitations which have been accepted. In the typical acceptability test for guidance, realism demands compromise because of limitations on the numbers and types of people available. However, it is possible to take precautionary steps that help avoid the more serious errors.

One approach that is suggested is to develop a roster of persons or groups of people who may be available for testing. In many cases, a roster of groups of people is maintained with some general demographics about the group. For any particular test, select respondents or groups from this roster by use of a random method. For any particular test, eliminate all persons who have in-depth knowledge of the product type or who have specific knowledge of the samples and variables being tested.

The use of persons in one's own company is problematic. If biases are likely because individuals receive free or reduced-price company products, "learn" the products by participating in tests frequently, or otherwise might know and select a product based not on the product's merits, but on other criteria, they should not be used.

Number of Respondents

The number of respondents is dependent on: the precision desired in the results, the risk of making an incorrect decision, and the representative of the people tested. However, a greater emphasis is placed on the last factor, representativeness.

Variability tends to be high in affective testing but is relatively constant for a given type of test. Precision (for example, in terms of the size of difference between treatments that one wants to be able to detect) often is a matter of arbitrary choice. Representativeness is related to the likelihood that the sample will be similar to some meaningful population. As more respondents are included, the possibility of selection bias may be reduced. Sampling within the usual limitations of population availability may not be technically possible, but compromises should be made only with the preceding factors in mind.

Some general guidelines in determining the number of respondents to be used are:

1. Conclusions based on results from small laboratory panels should be made with extreme caution and subject to further verification. Small laboratory panels, besides being too small to be representative of the larger population, often have biases related to products they use or encounter more frequently than the general consumer population. Bias related to knowledge about the product or sample or personal interactions with the testing staff are deterrents to this type of testing. However, panels numbering as few as 16 to 20 people are sometimes used, although the usual practice is to require at least 30. Even this number is small and represents only a rough screening. The error is large, and important trends can go undetected. Moreover, the representativeness of the people usually is questionable. However, this testing often is better than having a single researcher or group of managers make an arbitrary decision about a product.

2. Generally 100 people usually is considered adequate for most of the problems handled in small consumer tests, but the exact number depends on the experimental design. If properly selected, the respondents can be representative of the appropriate population. Experimental error usually will be small enough so that most important differences will be detected. (Note: Consumer testing for claims substantiation almost always requires larger numbers of respondents).

3. The use of larger numbers of respondents may improve the ability of the statistical procedures to "find differences," but may not do anything about possible biases in the population. For example, a large sample of company employees may be just as biased toward company products as a small sample. When the importance of the test objective, or of the decision that must be made, indicates the need for large tests, it is advisable to collect data from carefully chosen respondents.

4. It is extremely important to note that obtaining replicate judgments from a small group of respondents does not serve the same purpose as increasing the actual number of respondents. Such testing may reduce some experimental error, but does not correct for a limited scope of sampling.

Effects of Respondents on Interpretation of Results

Drawing unwarranted inferences and conclusions from test results is a serious fault that must be guarded against. A preference test made with an inadequate number of respondents, is not inherently wrong, *if* its limitations are recognized. For example, in a preference test where the number of respondents is small, it is possible to conclude that a preference exists if one is found, but it is not possible to conclude that the products are equally preferred if no preference is found. That limitation is based on the statistical power of the test. The problem in many consumer tests is that experimenters are prone to overlook the limitations in their zeal to report information. The limitations of a test must be recognized and reported if the results are to be useful.

Affective tests conducted with biased respondents are not only wrong, they can be extremely misleading. The possibility of potential biases in respondents leads to a strong cautionary statement. When the test is small or the sampling limited, pay particular attention to the possible effects of biasing factors. Do not generalize too broadly; recognize the limits of the test.

Orientation and Training of Respondents

Respondent orientation and training for analytical testing is designed to familiarize a respondent with test procedures, improve a respondent's ability to recognize and identify sensory attributes in complex product systems, and improve a respondent's sensitivity and memory so that he or she will provide precise, consistent, and standardized sensory measurements that can be reproduced. Training is not appropriate for affective testing, but it is appropriate to give some orientation to naive respondents (consumers) to help them understand the test.

Analytical Tests

Panel members must become thoroughly familiar with the tasks they will be expected to do. Respondents need a complete understanding of the nature of the judgments required, the test procedures, and the test controls that the respondent is required to maintain. The degree of training required will depend on the types of testing the respondents will perform.

Training may be continued through individual and group sessions in which various samples of the product types usually involved in the tests are evaluated and discussed. This is particularly important for respondents who will be required to make descriptive distinctions among products. For those tests it is necessary for all panel members to learn a common language.

Training should concentrate on the respondents' perceptual and judgmental tasks. The respondents do not need to understand test designs, mathematical treatment of data, and interpretation of results except what they need to know to understand feedback on their performance. Training respondents to recognize characteristics of a set of standards may help them disregard personal preferences and develop more stable judgments.

Under no circumstances should respondents in analytical tests be asked to make preference or acceptance judgments. Respondents in analytical tests are trained to disregard personal preferences. In addition they are trained to focus on specific characteristics and concentrate on all characteristics equally well in their analysis. Such training is necessary to provide good discriminating or diagnostic information about products. However, training also results in respondents who are no longer naive consumers. They no longer think about products as naive consumers do and must not be asked questions appropriate only for naive consumers to answer.

Affective Tests

Orientation should consist only of describing the mechanics of the test that the consumers (respondents) need to know. Any attempt to alter the respondents' attitudes or manner of arriving at decisions must be carefully avoided.

Incidental training on product characteristics such as specific off-flavors often is alleged to occur during continual testing. Although that probably does happen to a limited extent, there is no evidence that it is a serious problem within most testing programs. Of more concern is the potential bias of developing familiarity with a product during repeated testing so that new products introduced into tests are recognized as new and, therefore, "worse" than or "better" than, the traditional products. Where learning could bias the respondents, rotation of panel members on a staggered basis may help control over-testing by some respondents.

Motivation of Respondents

Obtaining useful results in any sensory test depends tremendously on maintaining a satisfactory level of motivation. The criteria for good motivation cannot be specific. However, poor motivation generally will be evidenced in hasty, careless testing, apparently poor discrimination, and a lessened willingness to participate.

Motivation is a complex area. People's behavior is caused by many factors that may interact in unpredictable ways. The most important thing is that the experimenter and management both recognize the importance of motivation, be aware of the conditions that affect it, and be alert for evidences of poor motivation.

One of the most important factors contributing to good motivation is interest in the test activity itself. With inexperienced respondents, who test only once or occasionally (for example, a short consumer study), interest usually is spontaneous, especially if they are compensated for their efforts either monetarily or otherwise. In the course of long-term panel work, interest may be reduced. Deliberate means, therefore, must be employed to motivate respondents.

For respondents who test frequently, whether they come from inside the organization or are "hired" expressly for this purpose, one of the best means of achieving good motivation is to maintain a high degree of status for the program and respondents. This can be achieved if the program is recognized as a useful and productive part of the respondents' work, if those in charge appear to know what they are doing, and if the tests are run efficiently. The respondents should be made aware of the importance of their contribution. A helpful practice is to publicize test results, whenever possible, without prejudicing future tests or compromising confidentiality. Adequate facilities and business-like laboratory procedures, maintained day after day, can develop respect for the program both from the respondents and from users and management. Favorable management attitudes are essential for a productive program. The positive reactions of management should be publicized sufficiently to favorably influence employee respondents or long-term respondents.

Other areas that contribute to motivation include pleasant physical and social surroundings and rewards. Money, products, prizes, or status are examples of rewards that are used in various testing programs.

Physiological Sensitivity of Respondents

Rules for maintaining physiological sensitivity cannot be specified in detail. Generally, they consist of avoiding conditions that might interfere with the normal functioning of the senses. Temporary adaptation from substances eaten or smelled usually are thought of as the major problems, but other problems may be overuse of muscles for texture or tactile phenomena or adaptation to light or color when visual stimulants are involved. Odor is particularly important, because respondents may become adapted to an odor continually present in the work place and remain unaware of the adaptation.

There is some evidence that physiological sensitivity fluctuates throughout the day; however, this time dependence apparently is not strong enough to preclude testing at any time during the normal working day. However, without evidence to the contrary the following are some general suggestions related to testing. Specific suggestions depend on the types of materials to be tested.

1. Wait to test for 1 h after meals or exercise to allow the body to return to some state of normality.
2. For food testing, wait at least 20 min after smoking, chewing gum, eating, or drinking. Encourage panel members to avoid eating highly spiced foods at the meal before they test to reduce carryover from previous oral stimulation.
3. For products such as textiles, the fingers and hands should be conditioned and maintained to prevent variations in the skin surface from affecting tests.
4. For testing of materials that depend on auditory or visual sensation, respondents should be instructed on techniques to prevent even short-term damage or adaptation by light or sound. The use of earphones and shifting the eyes over various surfaces or colors or both may be sufficient.
5. Do not use respondents who are ill or upset in any way because they may be physiologically unable to sense stimuli or be psychologically unable to concentrate on the testing task.
6. For any test where oral or nasal stimulation is to be measured, respondents should not use perfumed cosmetics and toiletries or lipstick. Respondents should wash their hands with odorless soap when they are required to handle containers or put their hands near the nose as part of testing.

One aspect of testing that must be considered is the elimination of the effects of the experimental samples themselves. Early samples in a series tend to adapt the senses and impact on later samples. With food, tastes and odors from previous samples may influence the following samples. With textile samples, lint from the samples may collect in the creases of the skin and reduce sensitivity. Assessment of color is partly dependent on visual adaptation with the previous sample. However, there are means of canceling or reducing the effects of a given sample.

With odor stimuli, normal breathing usually suffices if one waits 20 to 30 s. However, this is only a general guide. The time required will vary with the adapting stimulus; some substances may require considerably longer recovery periods and others may be shorter.

With taste stimuli, rinsing before the first sample and between subsequent samples with taste neutral water may be the best method. Certain products may require the use of reasonably bland foods such as unsalted crackers, celery, or apples to stimulate salivation and return to a neutral testing state. If such an agent is used it should be used prior to rinsing. Rinse water should be at room temperature, rather than cold. Water slightly above body temperature may be advisable when fatty foods are tested by trained respondents, but it should not be used in preference tests because of its generally unpleasant effect.

Rinsing between samples is not done universally. There is some evidence that subjects perform better in the triangle test if they follow the practice they prefer, either rinsing or not rinsing between samples.

Psychological Control

Sensory testing, whether analytical or affective, is concerned with the measurement and evaluation of stimuli by means of human behavior. Thus, the procedures outlined in this manual may be considered as an example of applied psychology. This does not mean that all operators need be trained in that science, nor that they must at all times consciously maintain the kinds of attitudes that are typically psychological in the clinical sense. However, it does mean that procedures must take into account the relevant psychological variables. One generally must be aware of the complexity of human behavior, learn how to deal with specific factors, and to anticipate and avoid sources of error and bias.

It would be impossible to list all possible psychological factors and dictate measures for their control; nor is it necessary. The same basic philosophy that applies to all experimental methods is applicable. Throughout this manual special procedures are described that incorporate elements of controlling psychological variables. They are particularly evident in the section on test methods, and many features of experimental design are directed toward the same purpose. The purpose of this section is to emphasize points that are considered particularly important and to list others that may not have been delineated elsewhere.

A respondent always reacts to the total situation. For example, in an affective test, a person's rating of a product reflects not only his feelings about the material but also many other factors, both transitory and permanent. Generally, those other factors are irrelevant to the purposes of the experiment. This is the reason for attempting to keep the experimental situation as constant as possible, keeping it quiet and comfortable, and eliminating outside pressures. Many features of test design and data analysis take this into account. For example, it is commonly accepted that comparisons between samples served to the same person in the same session often are more reliable than comparisons between samples served to different persons or to the same person at different times.

Cues

It is extremely important to remember that a respondent will use all available information in reaching a decision, even though he or she may know that it is irrelevant. This tendency, conscious or unconscious, is particularly important in the forced-choice sensory testing methods. A respondent may allow accidental variations in such things as sample size, containers, placement of samples, or other irrelevant information to influence the answer to the question asked in the test. This source of error usually can be avoided by rigorously adhering to the proper procedures of sample presentation. For example, it is ridiculous to present a set of samples that obviously are different in an attribute such as color to respondents in a triangle test and attempt to persuade them not to use that attribute to determine if the samples are different. The respondent knows that one product is different and believes he or she is expected to find that difference. Consequently, the difference will be found using the obvious differences as a cue. These tests should be conducted only if it is possible to mask the irrelevant differences.

Codes

Sensory testing usually seeks to evaluate the properties of a sample, apart from its developmental history. Thus, one must eliminate respondents who have special knowledge about the materials under test. Also, samples should be identified by code. However, the codes themselves may be biasing. For example, such code designations as A-1, X in relation to another letter, 1 as compared to 2, and many others are likely to have acquired meanings that could influence decisions. To reduce this source of error the following are important considerations:

1. Generally, use codes such as 3 digit numbers generated from a table of random numbers, that do not usually have an inherent meaning;
2. Use multiple codes for a sample even in a single session and over the course of many sessions;
3. Avoid the temptation to use a certain code, or set of codes, constantly to expedite tabulation of results.

Experimenter

It is a common phenomenon in psychological testing that respondents want to "please" the experimenters. They want to give "right" answers both to demonstrate their skills and to expedite, so they believe, the progress of science. This kind of cooperation must be avoided. Experimenters, particularly the operators who are giving instructions and presenting samples, must be aware of the possible effects of their own attitudes and even of chance statements. The proper approach is careful, impersonal neutrality. Avoid giving any hint of the expected results of an experiment, and do not discuss the samples with respondents prior to testing. Let them know that you are pleased to have them test (this is good for motivation) and let it appear that you will be no less pleased whatever the test results.

Bibliography

Amerine, M. A., Pangborn, R. M., and Roessler, E. B., *Principles of Sensory Evaluation of Food,* Academic Press, New York, 1965, Chapter 5, pp. 245–275.

Basker, D., "Comparison of Discrimination Ability Between Taste Panel Assessors," *Chemical Senses and Flavor,* Vol. 2, 1976, pp. 207–209.

Basker, D., "The Number of Assessors Required for Taste Panels," *Chemical Senses and Flavor,* Vol. 2, 1977, pp. 493–496.

Bennett, D. R., Spahr, M., and Dods, M. L., "The Value of Training a Sensory Test Panel," *Food Technology,* Vol. 10, 1956, p. 205.

Bressan, L. P. and Behling, R. W., "The Selection and Training of Judges for Discrimination Testing," *Food Technology,* Vol. 31, No. 11, Nov. 1977, pp. 62–67.

Chambers, E. IV, Bowers, J. A., and Dayton, A. D., "Statistical Designs and Panel Training/Experience for Sensory Analysis," *Journal of Food Science,* Vol. 46, 1981, pp. 1902–1906.

Coleman, J. A. and Wingfield, R., "Measuring Consumer Acceptance of Foods and Beverages," *Food Technology,* Vol. 18, No. 11, Nov. 1964, pp. 53–54.

Colwill, J. S., "Sensory Analysis by Consumer: Part 2," *Food Manufacture,* Vol. 62, No. 2, Feb. 1987, pp. 53–54.

Dawson, E. H., Brogdon, J. L., and McManus, S., "Sensory Testing of Difference in Taste: II Selection of Panel Members," *Food Technology,* Vol. 17, No. 10, Oct. 1963, pp. 39–44.

Gacula, M. C., Jr., Parker, L., and Kubala, J. J., "Data Analysis: A Variable Sequential Test for Selection of Sensory Panels," *Journal of Food Science,* Vol. 39, No. 6, June 1974, pp. 61–63.

Girardot, N. F., Peryam, D. R., and Shapiro, R. S., "Selection of Sensory Testing Panels," *Food Technology,* Vol. 6, 1952, pp. 140–143.

Hall, B. A., Tarver, M. G., and McDonald, J. G., "A Method for Screening Flavor Panel Members and Its Application to a Two Sample Difference Test," *Food Technology,* Vol. 13, No. 12, 1959, pp. 699–703.

Kramer, A., Cooler, F. W., Cooler, J., Modery, M., and Twigg, B. A., "Numbers of Tasters Required to Determine Consumer Preferences for Fruit Drinks," *Food Technology,* Vol. 17, No. 3, March 1963, pp. 86–91.

McDermott, B. J., "Identifying Consumers and Consumer Test Subjects," *Food Technology,* Vol. 44, No. 11, Nov. 1990, pp. 154–158.

Meilgaard, M., Civille, G. V., and Carr, B. T., *Sensory Evaluation Techniques,* 2nd ed., CRC Press, Boca Raton, FL, 1991, Chapter 4, pp. 37–42.

Mitchell, J. W., "Problems in Taste Difference Testing. I. Test Environment," *Food Technology,* Vol. 11, No. 9, Sept. 1957, pp. 476–477.

Nally, C. L., "Implementation of Consumer Taste Panels," *Journal of Sensory Studies,* Vol. 2, 1987, pp. 77–83.

Reynolds, A. J., "Sensory Analysis by Consumer: Part 1," *Food Manufacture,* Vol. 62, No. 1, Jan. 1987, pp. 37–38.

Shepherd, R., Griffiths, N. M., and Smith, K., "The Relationship Between Consumer Preferences and Trained Panel Responses," *Journal of Sensory Studies,* Vol. 3, 1988, pp. 19–35.

Stone, H. and Sidel, J. L., *Sensory Evaluation Practices,* 2nd ed., Academic Press, San Deigo, 1993, Chapter 4, pp. 99–106.

Thomson, D. M. H., *Food Acceptability,* Elsevier Applied Science, New York, 1988.

Wu, L. S., *Product Testing with Consumers for Research Guidance, ASTM STP 1035*, American Society for Testing and Materials, Philadelphia, 1989.

Wu, L. S. and Gelinas, A. D., *Product Testing with Consumers for Research Guidance: Special Consumer Groups, Second Volume, ASTM STP 1155*, American Society for Testing and Materials, Philadelphia, 1989.

Zook, K. and Wessman, C., "The Selection and Use of Judges for Descriptive Panels," *Food Technology*, Vol. 31, No. 11, Nov. 1977, pp. 56–61.

SAMPLES OF MATERIALS

Selection of Sample to be Tested

The problems of selecting materials for sensory testing are the same as selection for any other experimental or quality control purpose. The general principle is to select material that is representative of the product or process under study. Sometimes experimenters are concerned about selection of human respondents, but erroneously assume that the sampling of materials needs no attention.

One special caution related to the consequences of selecting samples from a single batch must receive attention. This is commonly done and must be considered carefully before proceeding with the test. If only one batch of product is made and tested, there is no information about the variation inherent in making that product, nor can one be sure that the product tested adequately represents the product that will be produced in subsequent batches. Obviously, however, the cost and time of producing additional batches must be considered. The point of this caution is not to preclude much of the testing that is conducted, but to be sure that the consequences of an action such as only producing a single batch, perhaps resulting in erroneous decisions, must be given due consideration.

Preparation of Samples

Procedures for preparing samples for testing must ensure that no foreign attributes are imparted unintentionally. Within a test, all samples should be prepared consistently with regard to factors that are subject to control.

In many instances there is freedom to select any one of a variety of methods of preparation for a given material. For example, tests of potatoes could be conducted with fried, boiled, mashed, baked, or even raw potatoes. Some important general factors are:

1. For difference testing, select the preparation method that is most likely to permit a detection of a difference if a variety of preparation methods are appropriate. Simplicity is the key. Generally, do not select preparations that may add competing flavors to samples, such as frying or the addition of seasoning. For fragrance testing, select an application method that will most likely result in total and even application of a controlled amount.

2. For preference testing, select a method that represents typical, normal use of the product. For example, a test of which closure is most useful for a bottle should be conducted on bottles of a size and shape that normally would be

encountered. Such testing helps ensure that the conditions for testing are similar to those found in use. For some products it is desirable to run tests using several different recipes. Often, preference test subjects are allowed to use such "voluntary" additions such as salt and pepper. However, the amount of those additions must be carefully controlled so that uniformity of addition is achieved for all samples. For example, if a respondent is allowed to add sugar to the first sample of coffee, the same amount (that is, pre-weighed in cubes or packets) must be added to each additional sample.

3. The question of the need for a "carrier" in preference tests often is pertinent. For example, do perfumes have to be applied to the skin for evaluation or does a study of frosting require it to be served on cake? This cannot be answered categorically. Valid comparisons among samples of many items can be made without using a normal carrier, but this depends on the nature of the material. Some materials (such as hot sauce, spices, and vinegar) require dilution because of their intense physiological effects. Each case must be decided on its own merits. Some materials must be tested on carriers the same as or similar to those they will be used with. For example, bittering agents, added to products to discourage children from swallowing them, must be tested in safe products or concoctions that are as similar as possible to the harmful materials because levels of addition must be determined and may vary tremendously from product to product.

Evaluation of materials (for example, food packaging) where the main question is whether tastes or odors will be imparted to other substances may require the special approach known as transfer testing, that makes use of flavor sensitive acceptor materials such as mineral oil, purified water, butter, chocolate, or foods that are typical of the contact foods. The test sample is placed in direct contact with the acceptor material for an appropriate time under appropriate conditions. For example, waxed packaging to be used at refrigerator or room temperature with fatty products may be made into a "sandwich" of two pieces of packaging with a butter center and placed in a bell jar for a period of 12 to 24 h. Control samples of the acceptor material are prepared by exposure under the same conditions except that the packaging material is absent. Samples of the acceptor material (butter in this example) are then tested both from those that have contacted the packaging material and those that have not. This approach may be used with a wide range of acceptor materials. Selection of the particular material and the conditions of exposure depend on the nature of the test sample and the conditions of its intended use.

Presentation of Samples

Samples should be presented in such a manner that respondents will react only on the basis of those factors which are intrinsic to the material tested. The key is uniformity within a given test and often from one test to another within a given product type. Important factors to consider are: quantity of sample, containers, temperature, and the special factors for the test such as the fabrics used to test fabric softeners, the apparatus for changing the viewing angle for paint finishes, or the eating utensils for food.

Amount of Samples

The amount of sample to be presented may vary over a considerable range. Usually, consideration of preparation effort, availability, and safety of materials set the upper limit. In difference tests, the criterion for the lower limit is to provide an amount sufficient to permit the average respondents to interact with the sample three times (that is, three "sips" or "bites" of a beverage or food or three "feels" for a fabric or paper test). Sometimes the test procedures may dictate a specific amount of sample. For example, respondents may be instructed to try each sample only once. In such instances, the quantity of sample can be adjusted accordingly.

It usually is not necessary, and often is distractive to provide full, normal quantities, even if the material is available, unless only one sample is to be tested. For example, it is easier to examine an automotive paint finish on a panel that can be manipulated easily than to show an entire car. Testing cake does not require that every respondent get a whole cake. From the respondents standpoint of view, testing full samples may be so overwhelming sensorially that there is difficulty sorting out the appropriate differences.

Some situations require whole products or entire samples to be presented. Limiting the sample size to only a few bits or a small area of skin application often is not appropriate, for example, in acceptability or preference tests conducted in the home, where normal consumption can be expected.

Temperature/Humidity Control in Sample Presentation

Whenever possible, samples should be presented at a temperature and humidity that is typical of normal consumption. Each test may have its own set of temperature or humidity requirements. Food usually is more dependent on temperature of serving while textiles may depend more on humidity. Fragrance products are dependent on both temperature and humidity. For affective testing the normalcy criterion becomes even more important. Whatever temperature or humidity is selected should be controlled and maintained throughout the test to provide consistent results.

Elimination of Appearance and Other Factors

Appearance factors come under the general topic of uniformity, but have a special feature. It sometimes is necessary to test samples for other sensory characteristics, even when they differ in appearance. Two brands of cookies or soap for example, may have characteristic differences that are difficult to obscure. For some types of tests to be conducted, differences must be eliminated by reducing illumination, using colored lights, using colored sample containers, the addition of a coloring, blindfolding respondents, or a combination of these.

Similarly, differences in other nonpertinent factors may be able to be masked by various means. For example, differences in conformation, texture, or consistency may be eliminated by subjecting all samples to maceration or blending. However this should be done only where such a change will not influence the attribute(s) under question. Blending, crushing, and other destructive methods must be avoided whenever texture is the issue, but also may need to be avoided for products such as fresh fruit or vegetables that can release enzymes upon cutting that would change the flavor, or for products such as soap where the change would alter bathing or ease of use.

Order of Presentation

When a test involves more than one sample, the order in which the samples are tested is very important. Respondents may react differently to the samples simply because of the order of presentation. This is related to the traditional "time error" of psychological experimentation. Also, they may react to a given sample differently because of the qualities of the sample that preceded it. This refers to "contrast effect" and "convergence effect." Experience has shown that no amount of instruction or training will avoid these effects completely without otherwise biasing results; nor is it necessary, since the effects can be understood and if not neutralized, at least explained as part of the test.

The principle is to balance the order of presentation among respondents so that over the entire test each sample will have preceded and followed each other sample an equal number of times. Such specific balancing often is not possible and it may be sufficient that each sample is tested in the first, second, third, or whatever position an equal number of times while randomly following the other samples. The same objective may be accomplished in a large experiment by randomizing order, but balancing provides more statistical objectivity. A statistician, or a person with this type of knowledge and experience, should be consulted whenever the design needs to deviate from simple or routine testing practices.

When samples are served simultaneously, as in triangle or rank order tests, the same problem exists. One sample must be considered before another. When samples can be received almost simultaneously, as in visual comparisons, the phenomenon is called "position error." The same solution applies here. Balance the geometric (for example, left to right) arrangement of samples, and give instructions to respondents for testing sequence so that over the entire experiment each sample is considered in each position, or time sequence, an equal number of times.

Number of Samples

The number of samples that should be presented in a given test session is a function of the type of product being tested and the "mind set" of the respondents. Obviously, the minimum number depends upon the test method. In most testing we are concerned with the maximum permissible number.

Generally, several samples or sets of samples may be considered during a single session. The actual number depends upon how quickly respondents may become fatigued or adapted. If the number of products is extended beyond a certain point, test results may show less discrimination. Strength of flavor, persistence of flavor, and anesthetic and other physiological effects all must be considered. Motivation is an important factor, as important as physiology. In many tests, respondents lose their desire to discriminate before they lose their physiological capability to do so.

Generally, it is permissible to conduct much longer sessions with trained respondents than with naive consumers (respondents). Here the experimenter, working constantly with the same group and, perhaps, the same materials, can adjust session length on the basis of feedback from the trained respondents and prior test results.

The "mind set" of the respondents cannot be over emphasized. Successful tests where consumers tested products for 4 h have been reported. It is common for trained panels to work from 1 to 3 h in a single test. The ability of respondents to do such long tests has as much to do with preparing the respondents for such testing before the test as it does with limiting adaptation to the stimuli. If respondents know they will be testing for extended periods, they generally are able to mentally prepare for the tests. Given appropriate spacing of samples and breaks in testing, respondents may do well in these extended sessions. Problems are encountered, however, when respondents believe they will be testing for only a specific period and the time exceeds that expectation. "Clock watching," day dreaming, and planning for the next activity take over quickly when expected testing time is exceeded, all to the detriment of good data.

The following recommendations are made as general guides to be used in the absence of more specific information about a particular test situation:

(a) When evaluating the acceptability of one type or class of products, three or four samples of most products may be presented. More can be tested if respondents expect the test to take a long time and adequate time is given between samples. Fewer samples must be presented if the samples cause sensory adaptation such as spicy foods or cloying perfumes.

(b) In paired comparison preference tests, three pairs often can be tested.

(c) In rank order tests, a maximum of four to six samples usually can be ranked. Although a larger number of samples may be tested, confusion in making comparisons often limits the number, except with visual stimuli where samples can be quickly compared.

(d) In evaluations of one type or class of products with trained panels, present no more than the panel feels capable of testing in a given time period. This often is two to six samples per hour depending on the length of the ballot.

In summary, sensory verdicts can be biased by a large number of factors, physiological as well as psychological. The use of a panel as an analytical instrument requires that all of these factors be avoided, or at least controlled.

TABLE 1—*Factors influencing sensory verdicts—physiological factors.*

Factors	Description	Examples
1. Adaptation	A decrease in or change in sensitivity to a given stimulus as a result of continued exposure to that stimulus or a similar one.	A respondent, having tested a set of soft drinks, is unable to properly score the sweetness in a less sweet sample.
2. Cross-adaptation	Adaptation caused by previous exposure to a different substance.	Insensitivity to the sweetness of sugar caused by previous exposure to another sweetener.
3. Cross-potentiation	Positive adaptation (or facilitation) caused by previous exposure to a substance of a different flavor.	An observer having been exposed to a sour candy perceives more sweetness in a subsequent sweet candy.
4. Enhancement	Effect of the presence of one substance increasing the perceived intensity of another presented simultaneously.	Amyl alcohols enhance the perceptions of the rose flavor of phenylethanol.
5. Synergy	Effect of the simultaneous presence of two or more substances increasing the perceived intensity of the mixture above the sum of the intensities of the components.	The impact on taste of monosodium glutamate is enhanced in mixtures with 5'ribonucleotides.
6. Suppression, masking	Effect of the presence of one substance decreasing the perceived intensity of another presented simultaneously.	Sweetness often suppresses or masks bitter or sour tastes. "A spoonful of sugar helps the medicine go down."

TABLE 2—Factors influencing sensory verdicts—psychological factors.

Factors	Description	Examples
1. Expectation error	Information deliberately or inadvertently supplied with the sample may trigger preconceived ideas.	A panelist hearing that an out-of-date product has been returned to the plant may tend to detect aged flavors in the day's test.
2. Error of habituation	Tendency to repeat the same response when samples show low levels of variation.	Respondents who continually test products that do not change may start to barely test the product and simply score the same, missing a difference in a new variation that was introduced.
3. Stimulus error	Observer is influenced by irrelevant criteria suggesting difference, such as the style or color of the container.	Wines in screw-capped bottles tend to be rated lower than wines in corked bottles.
4. Logical error	Observer modifies a verdict because two or more characteristics of the sample are associated in his mind.	A darker beer may be rated more flavorful. A darker mayonnaise may be rated more stale than it is.
5. Halo effect	Observer, having formed a low (or high) overall opinion of a sample, gives low (high) ratings to many attributes, including some which do not deserve this.	A fabric that receives a high overall rating also tends to be rated high on softness and cushiony, and low on rough, and scratchy, whether it has those characteristics or not.
6. Order of presentation effects		
a. Contrast effect	A sample, preceded by another of contrasting character, may receive a more extreme rating than if it had been evaluated monadically.	February 40°F weather in Minneapolis is a heat wave, in Miami it is a cold spell: a bland sample after a flavorful one may be rated blander than it would have if presented alone.
b. Group effect	One sample presented together with a group of samples of contrasting character may be rated closer to the group than if it had been evaluated alone.	A bland sample in the midst of many flavorful ones may be rated more flavorful.
c. Pattern effect	Panelists are quick to detect any repeated pattern in the order or manner of presentation of samples.	If flavorful samples often are served late in the test, panelists will return higher ratings for the flavor intensity of samples presented late.
d. Time error/positional bias	Subtle changes of attitude occur between the sample presented first and that presented last. The direction of this effect varies with circumstances.	In short tests the first sample may be rated higher because of anticipation of hunger or thirst; in long tests (for example, home placement) the last sample may be preferred.

7. Error of central tendency	Samples tend to be scored near the middle of the scale for fear that samples higher or lower will be encountered.	An extremely rancid potato chip may be scored as moderately rancid because the panelist is afraid that a more rancid sample will be tested.
8. Mutual suggestion	The response is influenced by other panelists' reaction.	Panelists frown, make comments, scratch their heads or taking longer or shorter than usual and influence other panelist responses.
9. Lack of motivation	Panelist takes less care than usual, or takes less care than other panelists.	Panelists who are doing the test not because they want to, but because they have to, may take less care to discern a subtle difference, search for a proper term, or be consistent in assigning scores.
10. Capriciousness versus timidity	Panelist exaggerates use of extremes of scale versus sticks to a narrow band in center of scale.	For the panelist who uses extremes, a minor decrease in crispness becomes extreme sogginess. For the panelist who always uses the same narrow band on the scale, substantial change from a shiny to a dull surface still results in only a minor change in scale.

Neglect of even one of them can spoil an investigation. Tables 1 and 2 are presented as a check list of sources of bias in sensory tests. It includes some sources already mentioned as well as additional ones to be considered.

Bibliography

Conner, M. T., Land, D. G., and Booth, D. A., "Effect of Stimulus Range on Judgments of Sweetness Intensity in a Lime Drink," *British Journal of Psychology,* Vol. 78, 1987, pp. 357–364.

Dean, M. L., "Presentation Order Effects in Product Taste Tests," *Journal of Psychology,* Vol. 105, 1980, pp. 107–110.

Eindhoven, J. and Peryam, D. R., "Measurement of Preferences for Food Combinations," *Food Technology,* Vol. 13, No. 7, July 1959, pp. 379–382.

Farley, J. U., Katz, J., and Lehmann, S. J., "Impact of Different Comparison Sets on Evaluation of a New Subcompact Car Brand," *Journal Consumer Research,* Vol. 5, No. 9, Sept. 1978, pp. 138–142.

Gacula, M. C., Jr., Rutenbeck, S. K., Campbell, J. F., Giovanni, M. E., Gardze, C. A., and Washam, R. W. II, "Some Sources of Bias in Consumer Testing," *Journal of Sensory Studies,* Vol. 1, 1986, pp. 175–182.

Gridgeman, N. T., "Group Size in Taste Sorting Trails," *Food Research,* Vol. 21, 1956, pp. 534–539.

Hanson, H. L., Davis, J. G., Campbell, A. A., Anderson, J. H., and Lineweaver, H., "Sensory Test Methods II. Effect of Previous Tests on Consumer Response to Foods," *Food Technology,* Vol. 9, No. 2, 1955, pp. 56–59.

Hutchinson, J. W., "On the Range Effects in Judgment and Choice," *Advances in Consumer Research,* Vol. 10, R. Bagozzi and A. Tybout, Eds., Association for Consumer Research, Ann Arbor, MI, 1983, pp. 305–308.

Kamen, J. M., Peryam, D. R., Peryman, D. B., and Kroll, B. J., "Hedonic Differences as a Function of Number of Samples Evaluated," *Journal of Food Science,* Vol. 34, 1969, pp. 475–480.

Kamenetzky, J., "Contrast and Convergence Effects in Rating of Foods," *Journal of Applied Psychology,* Vol. 43, 1959, pp. 47–52.

Kim, K. and Setser, C. S., "Presentation Order Bias in Consumer Preference Studies on Sponge Cakes," *Journal of Food Science,* Vol. 45, No. 4, 1980, pp. 1073–1074.

Kramer, A., Cooler, F. W., Cooler, J., Modery, M., and Twigg, B. A., "Numbers of Tasters Required to Determine Consumer Preference for Fruit Drinks," *Food Technology,* Vol. 17, No. 3, 1963, pp. 86–91.

Krik-Smith, M. D., Van Toller, C., and Dodd, G. H., "Unconscious Odour Conditioning in Human Subjects," *Biological Psychology,* Vol. 17, No. 2, 1983, pp. 221–231.

Kroll, B. J. and Pilgrim, F. J., "Sensory Evaluation of Accessory Foods with and without Carriers," *Journal of Food Science,* Vol. 26, 1961, pp. 122–124.

Laue, E. A., Ishler, N. H., and Bullman, G. A., "Reliability of Taste Testing and Consumer Testing Methods: Fatigue in Taste Testing," *Food Technology,* Vol. 8, 1954, p. 389.

Lynch, J. G., Jr., Chakravarti, D., and Mitra, A., "Contrast Effects in Consumer Judgments: Changes in Mental Representations or in the Anchoring of Rating Scales." *Journal Consumer Research,* Vol. 18, No. 3, Dec. 1991, pp. 284–297.

McBride, R. L., "Range Bias in Sensory Evaluation," *Journal of Food Technology,* Vol. 17, No. 2, 1982, pp. 405–410.

McBride, R. L., "Stimulus Range Influences Intensity and Hedonic Ratings of Flavour," *Appetite,* Vol. 6, 1985, pp. 125–131.

Sather, L. A. and Calvin, L. D., "The Effect of Number of Judgments in a Test on Flavor Evaluations for Preference," *Food Technology,* Vol. 14, No. 12, 1960, pp. 613–615.

Shepherd, R., Farleigh, C. A., and Land, D. G., "Effects of Stimulus Context on Preference Judgments for Salt," *Perception,* Vol. 13, 1984, pp. 739–742.

Chapter 2 — Forced Choice Discrimination Methods

The forced choice discrimination tests are used to confirm suspected small differences in product characteristics or product quality and to select respondents for discrimination tests. Sometimes discrimination is desirable, such as, with a planned improvement in a product versus the original. Sometimes discrimination is undesirable, such as, a change to a less costly ingredient or when trying to match the paint on a car door to the rest of the automobile after an accident. The tests given here are sensitive methods and, thus, are most applicable when the differences are slight. Paired comparisons and rating scales are more appropriate for large differences. Two major applications are in production quality control and cost reductions.

Several variants of discrimination tests are described. They have commonality in that each creates an arrangement of samples. The respondent is forced to choose one sample. This choice can either be designated as correct or incorrect. If the frequency of correct solutions is higher than that expected by chance, then a difference is declared.

If the number of correct responses is lower than that needed to declare the samples are different then it often is incorrectly stated that the samples are "the same." Traditional difference tests do not measure sameness; they are designed to measure difference. Although sometimes difficult to understand, a rejection of difference is not a measure of similarity. When the test is conducted properly and "difference" is not found we *infer* that the samples are similar, and often state "the same," but proof of similarity was not measured using these test methods. This distinction is especially important when small numbers of respondents are used, because we have low statistical power in the test and may incorrectly infer samples are the same when they were not. That is especially true of tests with difference tests with small numbers of respondents.

TEST TYPES

Triangular Test

In the triangular (often just called the triangle) test, three samples are presented simultaneously or sequentially. Two samples are the same and one sample is different. The respondent is asked to choose the "odd" sample. The triangle test has a statistical advantage over the paired comparison test when differences are small because respondents can guess correctly only one third of the time versus one half of the time in the paired comparison or duo-trio test.

Triangle Test: Case Study

Objective

Vitamin A fortification of milk is required by law, but higher levels of Vitamin A that are added to ensure legal compliance may result in flavor differences. Quality control has monitored both Vitamin A levels and complaints for the past year and believes problems are most prevalent at high Vitamin A levels. Thus, flavor tolerances for Vitamin A addition need to be established for quality control purposes. Quality control wants to ensure that no sensory differences are present in milk with the "control" or required Vitamin A level and milk with an upper limit of additional Vitamin A added.

Method

A triangle test was selected because an objective of "no difference" needed to be met. Thirty respondents, previously screened and known to be sensitive to Vitamin A flavor in milk, were recruited. All were familiar with triangle testing methodology. Instant milk was produced without any Vitamin A added. Vitamin A was added to samples of that batch to ensure that Vitamin A was the only varying factor. For the test, the control product was the target or required concentration. The concentration of Vitamin A added to the test product was the concentration of the upper rejection limit currently used by production.

Results

Sixteen correct judgments out of 30 were recorded. That is statistically significant at $p < 0.05$. (See Chapter 7, Table 3b).

Recommendations

The upper limit is too high for people sensitive to the Vitamin A flavor. Additional testing is necessary to determine an upper production limit that does not produce a product different between the control and the target product.

Duo-Trio Test

In the duo-trio test the set of samples is the same as in the triangle test, but, one of the matched samples is identified as the "reference." The reference sample always is considered first. The respondent is directed to determine which of the other two samples is the same as the reference. Usually, the samples are presented simultaneously, but they can be presented successively.

Duo-Trio Test: Case Study

Objective

An alternate supplier is needed for a spice blend used in a salsa product currently on the market. The product should retain its present profile; no difference in the product is desirable.

Method

The duo-trio test method was chosen because the product has a high flavor impact and medium burn. The duo-trio requires two taste comparisons where the triangle would require three to reach the decision. Also, because a single attribute, such as "burn," is not important, but rather the entire product is important, a paired difference is not appropriate.

Products were manufactured using the current and proposed spice blends. They were made using common ingredients on the same day. Eighteen respondents were recruited from a respondent pool of discriminators, experienced in testing tomato based products.

Results

Ten correct responses out of 18 were obtained. As 13 correct judgments would be required to show a significant difference at $p < 0.05$, we conclude that proof of difference was not found and accept the alternate supplier (Chapter 7, Table 2). (*Note:* In this case, the "risk" associated with accepting an alternate supplier that was not exactly the same was low. Thus the company decided they could use a reasonably small number of respondents for the duo-trio test. The company increased its risk of finding no difference when a difference might really have existed by using a small number of respondents. They reduced risk somewhat by using respondents who were known discriminators.)

3-Alternative Forced Choice Test

The 3-alternative forced choice (3-AFC) test is a variant of the triangle test where the same sample always is used as the matched pair. The 3-AFC test is most often used when the samples vary in strength, but not character. The sample that is suspected to be stronger almost always is used as the single or "different" sample. In addition, instead of asking panelists to select the odd sample or the pair, they are asked to select the "stronger" sample. The 3-AFC test eliminates perceptual problems that can arise when the sample that is "stronger" is used as the pair. The data analysis is similar to the triangle test.

3-Alternative Forced Choice Test: Case Study

Objective

Cost reduction is necessary to maintain profit margins on a currently marketed fabric softener. One cost savings is to reduce the level of fragrance added to the fabric softener. The actual fragrance is not to be changed, but a 20% reduction is needed. Research and Development and Marketing want to be sure that no difference is found, if the fragrance level is reduced.

Method

A difference test was selected because an objective of "no difference" needed to be met before reduction in fragrance could occur. The 3-AFC procedure was used because only a change in intensity, not character of the fragrance, was expected to occur if any difference was noted.

Two fabric softeners were produced, one with the current level of fragrance and one with a reduced level. A typical triangle test setup was used, but the test product with less fragrance was always used as the pair and panelists were asked to find the "stronger" sample. Those "changes" to the triangle test made this into a 3-AFC procedure.

In addition, the company wanted to be reasonably sure that they found a difference in fragrance strength if one existed. Therefore, they selected the 10% probability level rather than the usual 5% to reduce the chance of not finding a difference if one existed. They used 40 screened panelists who were known to be discriminators.

Results

Nineteen of 40 panelists correctly selected the stronger sample. Using Chapter 7, Table 3a, the researchers found that 18 of 40 was needed for a significant difference and, therefore, concluded that a difference had been found and the 20% reduction in fragrance was too much to maintain the integrity of the current product.

A recommendation to test a lower reduction in fragrance level (for example, 10%) was made and also to determine additional mechanisms for reducing cost.

Paired Difference Test

Paired difference tests are used to find if a difference exists for some specified attribute. Two samples are presented, either simultaneously or sequentially, and the respondent chooses one of the samples as having a higher level of some specified characteristic. For example, "Which sample is sweeter, smoother, whiter, etc." The specified characteristic or attribute must be commonly understood by all respondents and may require a standard or reference to illustrate the character. The most common use of paired difference is the "preference test" where the attribute question essentially becomes "which sample is preferred."

Paired Difference Test: Case Study

Objective

Consumer testing indicated a new cheese sauce is too sour. The product has been reformulated to reduce sourness. Informal bench-top screening indicated that the sourness has been reduced. Sensory testing will be run to verify the results.

Method

A paired difference test to determine which of two samples (current "new" cheese sauce or reformulated "new" cheese sauce) is less sour is conducted. This test was chosen over a triangle or duo-trio test in order to focus on the single attribute of sourness. Management has accepted the fact that other sensory parameters likely will be affected by a reduction in sourness.

Twenty-five respondents were chosen from the laboratory respondent pool. Red lights were used to eliminate any possible visual differences and respondents practiced testing under red lights so that the "strange" lighting did not affect panelist performance. Respondents were instructed to rinse between samples with room temperature water.

Results

Eighteen of the 25 respondents selected the reformulated product as less sour. That number of responses is significant at $p < 0.01$; thus, the reformulated product is perceived to be less sour than the current product. The test is a one-tailed test (Chapter 7, Table 2) because it was known by researchers which of the products should be less sour.

Recommendations

Having met the goal of reformulation, a new sensory profile or description of the product needs to be established and the sample resubmitted for consumer testing.

A-not-A Test

This test is designed for a special type of difference testing problem, where the "standard" cannot be represented by a single product. For example, fresh vegetables vary from piece to piece even if they are of the same variety and grown on the same plant. Triangular or duo-trio tests could show differences from one tomato to another even grown on the same plant. Thus, most commonly used difference tests often are not useful for studying differences from variety to variety. The typical question in an A-not-A test is whether a test set or lot of product differs from the product type it should represent.

The respondent is required to study "control" materials until he or she believes either can identify the control consistently. Other materials also may be examined by the respondents to understand what differences may be present. The respondent then is presented with a series of control and experimental samples, the order of which has been determined randomly and is required to identify the samples as "control" or not. In other words, "A" or "not A." This method is useful only when the "control" sample can be recognized as the control or standard product even though it may have some variation. The number of "A's" and "not-A's" in the test usually is the same and usually varies from two to five of each. (See Meilgaard et al. for more information and analysis of this test).

Multiple Standards Test

This test is designed for a special type of problem, where the standard cannot be represented by a single product. The typical question is whether a test lot of product differs generically from a product type within which there is, or may be, considerable variability. For example, in testing products such as multicomponent soups or cereals it is difficult to determine if samples are different or not because each "bite" may have a slightly different number of vegetables, meat bits, nuts, flakes, etc. Similarly, different pilot plant productions of a paper product, such as tissues, may have variations even when made according to the same specifications. The problem in these cases is not to find the different product, because all of the products, even the "same" products may test "different" from each other. Rather the issue is to find the product that is more different from all the others.

In that respect the multiple standards test is similar to the "A-not-A" test. However, in the multiple standards test, the respondent is not required to "learn" the control samples before the test begins, a time savings. One limitation of the multiple standards tests is that it limits the respondents' knowledge of product variation to those variations that are in the "test set," without benefit of knowing about other natural variations in the product that could be present. For products where considerable batch to batch variation is not present this test is quite effective. However, when it is possible to "learn" a product, for example, smokers may know a "brand," the appropriate test probably is the A-not-A test.

Several (preferably two to five) "blind" standards representing the product type and one "blind" test product are presented to the respondent, and he or she is instructed to select the sample which differs most from all of the others. The multiple standards test may work well even when control products do not match exactly, and the respondent is allowed to select the sample that is most different.

The statistic for the test is based on the number of times the "test" sample is selected as most different. The exact statistic is calculated based on a binomial distribution for the number of samples in the test. For example, if three standards and one test product are included, the statistic is calculated using a null hypothesis probability of $p = 1/4$ because the chance of selecting the test sample when no overall difference exists is 1 out of 4.

The statistic often is calculated by approximating the binomial distribution using the z-score. Suppose $n = 30$ respondents participated in a multiple standards test with $s = 3$ standard sample and one test sample. If $x = 12$ respondents selected the test sample as being the most different, then the z statistic is calculated as:

$$z = \frac{x - n(p_0)}{\sqrt{n(p_0)(1 - p_0)}} = \frac{12 - 30(1/4)}{\sqrt{30(1/4)(1 - (1/4))}} = \frac{4.50}{2.37} = 1.897$$

where $p_0 = 1/(s + 1)$, s being the number of standard samples in the test. The test statistic z follows a standard normal distribution. The critical values of the standard normal are the same as those of the Student's t distribution with ∞ degrees of freedom. Entering the last row of the Student's t table, Chapter 7, Table 4, one finds that $z = 1.645$. Therefore, it is concluded that the test sample in this example is significantly different from the standards.

Multiple Standards Test: Case Study

Objective

A soup manufacturer is considering reducing the salt by 25% in "chunky" vegetable soup. Products are made both with the standard level and the reduced level of salt and sent for difference testing.

Method

Originally, the sensory analyst considered having each person make sure that each bite contained some of each ingredient but quickly realized that was not possible with this product. Next, the analyst considered testing each component (for example, beef broth, potato, carrot, peas) separately, but realized that the sensory effects found in individual ingredients would not represent actually eating the soup. Because testing of this product was done infrequently, having participants "learn" many natural variations of the product in each bite were considered unnecessary and impractical. Thus, a multiple standards test was selected.

Thirty-two panelists were selected from the pool of known discriminators and were served four samples. One sample was the reduced salt product and three samples were the currently marketed products. For this test the three samples were different lots of production. (NOTE: different lots are not required for this test although having different lots provides more "real" variation in the study).

Results

Fourteen of the 32 panelists correctly selected the reduced salt product as the "most different" sample in the set. The z-score was calculated ($z = 2.45$) and compared to the t-statistic (1.64) for infinity degrees of freedom for the 5% level, one-tailed test (Chapter 7, Table 4). Because z exceeded that value we conclude that the reduced salt formula was noticeably different from the control.

Recommendations

Based on the results from this test, the lower salt soup cannot be substituted for the standard soup without reformulation. Descriptive studies may be needed to determine how the products differ in order to give specific reformulation help to the product developers. Management may determine that the salt reduction is important enough to sales to reduce the salt even though the product is different, but in that case other tests, such as affective guidance tests and marketing studies, need to be conducted to determine whether the product will continue to be successful if salt is reduced.

Design of Difference Tests

Certain basic features of experimental design apply to the forced choice methods just as with any other method. For example, it is necessary to balance sample presentation to control for time or position error. However, certain special problems also arise with tests of this type.

With both the triangle test and the duo-trio test it is necessary to determine for any given test which of the two samples should be given as the pair and which should be the "different" sample. This can be done in two ways. Either one of the samples can be selected for use as the reference or pair throughout the whole test (this is the 3-AFC test when done in triangle testing), or the two samples can be used alternately as the reference or pair. Which procedure to adopt should be decided by the following.

1. When one has no knowledge about the possible differences, it generally is better to use the two samples alternately as the reference or pair. It is a good idea to present all six combinations (ABB, BAB, BBA, BAA, ABA, AAB) in a random pattern until the needed sample size is obtained in a triangle test. Likewise, all four combinations would be presented in a duo-trio test (Reference = A, Presentation = A, B; Reference = A, Presentation = B, A; Reference B, Presentation = A, B; Reference = B, Presentation = B, A). Respondents may anticipate a particular sequence. Thus, the respondents should not be aware of how the sequences are established.

2. There are several cases where it is advantageous to use the same reference or matched pair throughout because it increases the probability of discrimination by reducing perceptual problems and biases.

(a) Respondents often are more likely to discriminate when the reference represents a familiar perceptual experience rather than a strange or new one. For example, that situation occurs when one wants to determine whether a process variation or a formula change with a standard product has changed its flavor appreciably. If respondents are familiar with the standard product and have tested them many times a change may be "strange" or "new." In that case, the standard product generally is used as the pair or the reference product. An analogous situation is where production samples are being checked against an accepted standard. In cases such as this, the well-known standard product often is selected as the reference.

(b) Respondents often are more likely to discriminate when the different sample is more intense than the matched samples. Hence, the less intense sample should be used as the reference or the matched pair whenever it is known, or suspected, that the major difference between the samples will be in regard to intensity. For example, one may want to determine a tolerance for the addition of a strong-flavored ingredient to a product. Here one would use the sample with the lesser amount of the ingredient as the reference or matched pair.

When a respondent is to be given two or more forced choice tests in immediate succession, it is necessary to control for what may be called "expectation" effects. The respondent may expect the position or time sequence of the samples in the tests to bear some logical relation to those in earlier tests. For example, if he or she judged the first unknown to be the "different" sample in the first of the duo-trio tests, he or she might expect the second unknown to be the "different" sample in the second test. Normal control procedures for time error or position error dictate that each possible sequence or pattern of positions should be used equally often in the course of a given test. To control for expectation effect, it is important that the allocation of sequences or patterns for each respondent be done randomly and that the respondents are aware that this is so.

The A-not-A tests present a special problem of expectation effect, because the longer the series, the more likely it is that respondents will divert their attention from finding A or not A to trying to "figure out" the series. The respondent may decide that (1) the experimenter will alternate the control and experimental samples or (2) that after a certain number of controls, the next sample will be an experimental sample, or (3) that exactly the same number of control and experimental samples will be given during the series. The identity of each sample in the sequence must be determined randomly and independently. However, from a statistical standpoint it is best to have the same number of control and experimental samples. Respondents should not be given that information, but the sequences should be determined with that in mind. Again, respondents should be made aware that the sequences are randomly established to help reduce expectation errors.

Sample Size

The number of tests can be determined statistically by choosing the alpha (α) and beta (β) risk levels and the difference that it is important to detect (see Chapter 7 on Statistics). Twenty to 40 comparisons often are made in the triangle test. If this number of comparisons is made for each respondent then the proportion of respondents finding a difference can be estimated. Guidelines on the number of samples that should be tried by a respondent in a single session were set forth earlier.

Difference tests often are used in relatively constant situations where the same type of material is tested by the same respondents over a long period. This permits experimentation with the system to determine how far the maximum number of tests may be extended. The limits will depend on the type of material to be tested, the training and motivation of the respondents, and the extent to which one may be willing to sacrifice discrimination in the interests of the economy of testing. This may be especially useful in quality control applications when the number of available respondents is small. Running multiple tests in a row on the same respondents should not be adopted without first experimentally showing their feasibility in the particular situation in which they are to be used.

Method Selection

No single test type is appropriate in all situations. For a given situation, selection of a discrimination method should be based on the objective of the test and the nature of the test product. The triangle and 3-AFC tests are statistically more sensitive than the duo-trio test because the chance of guessing the correct response is 1/3 rather than 1/2. However, because the triangle test and the 3-AFC also are more likely to produce adaptation from more frequent testing (that is, tasting, smelling, rubbing the sample) or may be more confusing psychologically because of the need to keep in mind the attributes of three unknowns rather than two unknowns, it is suggested that no one method be considered superior under all conditions.

Extensions of Difference Test: Complex Sorting Tasks

All forced-choice methods may be considered as "sorting-tasks" even the paired difference test which requires only the sorting of two objects into two classes. The essence of the methods described previously is simplicity. Tasks of increasing complexity can be designed readily. For example, the respondent may be presented with eight samples, four of one kind and four of another, and asked to sort them into their two classes. Usually the merit alleged for such tests is their efficiency in the sense that the probability of a fully correct solution by chance alone is very low; hence, a difference can be proven with only a few trials. However, it is also true that, as complexity increases, so also does the probability that a respondent will make errors even though he or she may have the proven capability of determining the difference between the products. More-over, the frequent failures associated with such tests tend to affect motivation adversely. Thus, although complex sorting tasks are valid for experimenting on perception and problem solving, the more simple test forms should almost always be used for regular, product-oriented work.

Interpretation of Results

The usual analysis of forced-choice data is to compare the observed number of correct responses with the number that theoretically would result from chance alone and to calculate the probability of the occurrence of the observed number. If that probability is low, we say that a difference has been established. One is more certain of a result at the 5% risk level than of one at the 10% risk level. However, it is not valid to consider these levels of significance as a measure of the degree of difference between products because the probability is critically dependent on the number of trials.

Difference tests often are run with a small number of trained screened respondents under specialized test conditions. When this is true, we cannot project that a difference detected by the respondents will be detected by the typical consumer, but only that it is possible. On the other hand, when the test has been conducted with an adequate number of screened respondents, a "no-difference" result provides reasonably good assurance that the consumer will not find a difference.

SPECIAL CASES OF FORCED-CHOICE DIFFERENT TESTING

Forced-Choice Difference Test: Degree of Difference

Although a commonly used procedure, it generally is inappropriate to ask a degree of difference rating following a forced-choice difference test such as the triangle test. Researchers often want to know if the difference is large or small. That decision should help in selecting the test. If the difference is expected to be small, a difference test should be used and "no degree of difference" test is necessary. If the degree of difference may be large, a forced choice difference test is inappropriate and a degree-of-difference test should be used from the start.

Forced Choice Difference Test: Characterization of Difference

This is a special purpose variant of the triangle test designed to provide a description of the perceived difference. The respondents are asked to identify or describe the characteristics that distinguish the samples perceived as identical from the sample perceived as different. The method is useful only as a qualitative bench top screening technique. Its primary advantage is to determine the need for an additional test, subsequent to the basic triangle test, to characterize the nature of the difference. However, this method often is abused. If difference test respondents have not been trained in descriptive methods, they likely are not able to reliably "name" the difference. Often they give answers that are misleading because their descriptive vocabulary is not well developed. Data from such respondents tend to be scattered and, generally, should not be used.

If the respondents have had descriptive training, the descriptions, only from those respondents who got the correct answer on the forced-choice test, can be sorted into similar/like categories and then reviewed for possible trends. One problem, even with respondents who have had descriptive training is that some percentage of the respondents are expected to get the correct answer by guessing; thus, data from some respondents (which ones are not known) are counted from respondents who just guessed the correct sample.

Forced-Choice Difference Test: Preference Test

The difference test followed by a preference test is occasionally done and should be discouraged. The two types of tests have a completely different psychological basis and usually are conducted with different types of respondents. Difference tests normally should be conducted with respondents selected for their ability to discriminate and preference tests are conducted with naive respondents (consumers) who represent the target market. Even when the respondents used for the two tests are similar, using the preference information only from those respondents who get the difference test correct is problematic. It is impossible to separate respondents who get the difference test correct merely by guessing who from those respondents actually discriminated. Therefore when a preference test is allowed after the discriminative test the preference results of people who guess correctly are mixed with those who really found differences. It is better to separate the difference tests from the preference test and treat each independently.

Bibliography

Brud, W., "Simple Methods of Odor Quality Evaluation of Essential Oils and Other Fragrant Substances," *Perfume Flavorist,* Vol. 8, 1983, pp. 47–52.

Francois, P. and Sauvageot, F., "Comparison of the Efficiency of Pair, Duo-Trio and Triangle Tests," *Journal of Sensory Studies,* Vol. 3, No. 2, 1988, pp. 81–94.

Frijters, J. E. R., "The Effect of Duration of Intervals Between Olfactory Stimuli in the Triangular Method," *Chemical Senses,* Vol. 2, 1977, pp. 301–311.

Frijters, J. E. R., "Variations of the Triangular Method and the Relationship of Its Unidimensional Probabilistic Models to Three-Alternative Forced-choice Signal Detection Theory Models," *British Journal of Mathematical and Statistical Psychology,* Vol. 32, 1979, pp. 229–241.

Frijters, J. E. R., Blauw, Y. H., and Vermaat, S. H., "Incidental Training in the Triangular Method," *Chemical Senses,* Vol. 7, No. 1, 1982, pp. 63–69.

Hall, B. A., Tarver, M. G., and McDonald, J. G., "A Method for Screening Flavor Panel Members and Its Application to a Two Sample Difference Test," *Food Technology,* Vol. 13, No. 2, Dec. 1959, pp. 699–703.

MacRae, A. W. and Geelhoed, E. N., "Preference Can Be More Powerful Than Detection of Oddity as a Test of Discriminability," *Perception Psychology,* Vol. 51, No. 2, 1992, pp. 179–181.

Mitchell, J. W., "Effect of Assignment of Testing Materials to the Paired and Odd Position in the Duo-Trio Taste Difference Test," *Food Technology,* Vol. 10, No. 4, April 1956, pp. 169–171.

Peryam, D. R. and Swartz, V. M., "Measurement of Sensory Differences," *Food Technology,* Vol. 5, 1950, pp. 207–210.

Peryam, D. R., "Sensory Difference Tests," *Food Technology,* Vol. 12, No. 5, May 1958, pp. 231–236.

Roessler, E. B., Pangborn, R. M., Sidel, J. L., and Stone, H., "Expanded Statistical Tables for Estimating Significance in Paired-Preference, Paired-Difference, Duo-Trio and Triangle Tests," *Journal of Food Science,* Vol. 43, 1978, pp. 940–947.

Thieme, U. and O'Mahony, M., "Modifications to Sensory Difference Test Protocols: The Warmed Up Paired Comparison, the Single Standard Duo-Trio, and the A-not A Test Modified for Response Bias," *Journal of Sensory Studies,* Vol. 5, No. 3, 1990, pp. 159–176.

Chapter 3—Scaling

Scaling methods are based on the respondent giving a value that indicates the type or intensity of a response. A dimension of evaluation must be specified; for example, a product characteristic or attribute. Scales need not be numerical. Graphic lines or other methods of measuring intensity or order may be used by respondents to specify their perceptions. Nonnumerical scales usually are converted to numerical values for purposes of statistical analysis.

Scales traditionally have been classified as producing data in one of four major divisions: nominal, ordinal, interval, and ratio.

(a) Nominal data define the type or category of a perception and does not indicate a quantitative relationship among categories. Frequently, nominal data are used to define respondents in terms of categories (such as gender, age, or user affiliations) where no relative merit can be assigned to the categories. Specifying whether an attribute is "present" or "not present" in a product is, in essence, a nominal scaling procedure. It must be noted that some people do not classify the collection of nominal data as scaling, although it is so classified in much of the psychological literature.

(b) Ordinal data identify relationships on a "more" or "less" basis. An example of ordinal scaling is "ranking" or "rank-order" testing. Scaling that produces ordinal data requires that two or more (generally three or more) objects be arranged in ascending or descending order based on the intensity, quantity, or size of some specified characteristic. Ordinal data often are used to screen a series of samples to detect outliers or other products that do not need more thorough investigation. Preference testing, that is, determining which of two samples is more preferred, probably is the most common scaling task resulting in ordinal data.

(c) Interval data consist of successive, equal-interval units that indicate the magnitude (generally intensity) of a product characteristic. The units arbitrarily are assigned numbers (often beginning at 0 or 1) that increase as the degree of magnitude increases. Frequently, scales that produce interval data are anchored at various points (usually the low and high end and, sometimes, the midpoint) with terms that indicate the magnitude of a response. Because of their flexibility, interval-type scales are used extensively in "descriptive analysis" to determine the intensity of a specified attribute. The data from scales used in studies that determine degree of like/dislike for a product often are treated as interval data for statistical purposes, although they probably produce ordinal data because the scale intervals may not be equal.

(d) Ratio data (magnitude estimation is the most common) indicates the magnitude of response and also specifies the relative ratio relationship of two or more responses. Numbers (or other measures) are assigned that reflect ratio differences between products. Scales that yield ratio data have been used in tests such as those described for interval scaling. However, these scales appear to be most

38

useful when studying the relationships of single sensory characteristics to physical stimuli, such as the relationship of sweetness and sugar concentration. All scaling methods have broad application. Any perceptual dimension that can be conceptually understood and quantified can be scaled. In sensory applications the nature of the stimuli can vary widely as can the perceptual dimension. For example, a food substance may be measured for sweetness intensity or degree of hardness; floor polishes may be studied for characteristics of gloss or translucency; and antiperspirants or deodorants must be evaluated for their own fragrance properties as well as their control of mal-odor. Scales are useful to measure attitudes, feeling, or opinions in many situations.

Rating Scales

All rating scale methods, usually interval or ratio in nature, provide the respondent with a dimension to evaluate and a scale showing order of magnitude. Stimuli (for example, food samples, hand lotions, or facial tissues) are presented, and the respondent's task is to assign each product a scale value to reflect the amount or intensity of the specified attribute. Multiple attributes usually are evaluated for each product.

Rating scales have broad application. In theory, they can be used with any psychological dimension that can be perceived, is quantifiable, and can be conceptually understood. In the sensory applications with which this manual is concerned, the evaluation is based on the respondent's immediate perception of a stimulus or his feelings about that stimulus, although rating scales also can apply to feelings or opinions in more general situations. Common applications of rating scales include:

1. Evaluation of hedonics (liking), that is, "likes" and "dislikes."

2. Evaluation of the degree or intensity of specific attributes of a material, such as sweetness, hardness, redness, roughness, or amount of off-flavor in food; or roughness, scratchiness, translucency, oiliness, wetness, or resiliency of a wet wipe.

3. Evaluation of respondents' opinions about the quality or degree of excellence of materials.

4. Evaluation, in either hedonic or quality terms, of the response to certain general attributes of a product, such as texture, appearance, flavor, or efficacy. NOTE: remember that the use of such general terms as "texture" frequently provides little specific information about a product. Also, it may be difficult for most people to describe their liking for one attribute independent of other attributes. For example: a consumer who does not like the "texture" of a cake also may indicate that he or she dislikes the flavor, even if the flavor is not objectionable.

In basic scope, rating scale methods cover almost the same applications as paired comparisons and rank order; there is a great deal of overlap in their application. However, rating scales give different information than paired comparison or rank order methods because they imply specific intensities of product attributes rather than just ordinal comparisons. That feature of rating scales produces certain inherent considerations for using such scales. Respondents must exercise a greater degree of sophistication in describing attribute intensities than they do with rank order. Further, it must be possible for the experimenter to describe, and for the respondent to perceive, more than two degrees of the attribute measured if it is to have advantages over paired comparison or rank order.

Rating scales may be used in test situations where samples of a series are presented simultaneously or in sequence. Regardless of presentation, the order in which the samples are tested should be controlled by instructions and based on sound statistical design principles.

Types of Rating Scales

A notable feature of rating scales is the great variety of particular scales that have been and are being used. The central idea of a rating scale is to create a continuum of some unidimensional concept and provide the respondent a means of locating an object in a position on that continuum. The following types of scales are used frequently:

Graphic Scale—These scales consist of either a simple line or one marked off into segments. The direction of the scale, that is, which end is "good" and which is "bad" or which is "high" and which is "low" must be shown clearly. Often, the intensity is established as a left to right reading continuum with low or bad on the left side and high or good on the right side of the page. However, many people use a right to left continuum to obtain equally good data. Also, that left/right or top/bottom continuum may need to be changed in cultures where top to bottom, left to right reading is not standard.

Examples:

Mark the appropriate point on the line (or check a box):

none   high

NONE ☐ ☐ ☐ ☐ ☐ ☐ ☐ ☐ ☐ HIGH

DISLIKE   NEITHER LIKE   LIKE

EXTREMELY   NOR DISLIKE   EXTREMELY

Verbal Scale—These scales consist of a series of brief written statements, usually the name of the dimension with appropriate adverbial or adjectival modifiers, that are written out in appropriate order.

Example:

Place a check next to the appropriate statement:

Like Extremely	————
Like Very Much	————
Like Moderately	————
Like Slightly	————
Neither Like nor Dislike	————
Dislike Slightly	————
Dislike Moderately	————
Dislike Very Much	————
Dislike Extremely	————

Numerical Scale—These scales consist of a series of numbers ranging from low-to-high, that are understood to represent successive levels of quality or degrees of a characteristic.

Examples:

Circle the number that describes the intensity:

None 0 1 2 3 4 5 6 7 8 9 10 11 12 13 14 15 Strong Extremely

Or the original Flavor Profile Scale:

) (= threshold
1 = slight
2 = moderate
3 = strong

Scale of Standards—The distinguishing feature of these scales is the frequent use of actual physical samples of material (references) to represent the scale categories. Sometimes such scales are partial; some but not all of the scale categories are represented by physical standards. Often, these scales are numerical scales and have references that represent a specific numerical value on the scale.

NOTE: Many verbal, numerical or line scales can have references or standards marked on the scale and may be considered scales of standards.

Example: Hardness (foods)

Scale Value	Product	Type/Brand	Manufacturer/ Distributor	Sample Size	Temperature
1.0	cream cheese	Philadelphia	Kraft	1/2 in. cube	40 to 45°F
6.0	olive	stuffed, Spanish type, pimento removed	Goya Foods	1 piece	room
11.0	almond	Planter, shelled	Nabisco Brands	1 piece	room

Pictorial Scales—These scales consist of pictures that represent the various degrees of the attribute or attitude. The most famous of these scales are "smiling faces" although size or number of stars, or other pictorial representations can be used.

Examples:

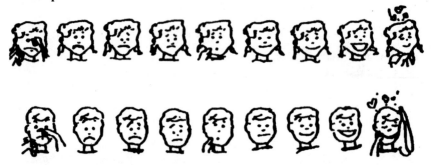

Length of Scale Formats

The length of each of the scales may vary. Physical extent may vary within wide limits without affecting results as long as the scale remains easy to read. While an exact recommendation regarding the number of segments or points which are specifically designated on the scale is not justified, certain guides may be provided.

1. Graphic, unstructured line scales are dependent on length of the line or the space the scale occupies and may be physically measured with a ruler or by computer. In general, graphic scales are considered to have more equal-interval properties than verbal or numerical scales, but graphic scales may not be appropriate in some situations.

2. Rating scales usually should not have fewer than five categories. Some special scales, such as "just about right" scales, may have only three categories,

such as "too little", "just right", or "too much," but those are exceptions that should be used carefully. Also, most liking rating scales have an odd number of categories in order to provide a midpoint that often is assumed to be "neutral." Odd-numbers of categories are not needed for intensity scales because they do not have midpoints.

3. For acceptance or liking scales the number of categories usually is balanced for like and dislike. The tendency to use unbalanced scales, that is, more like categories than dislike categories, on the supposition that most products are good, should be avoided. First, the researchers' assumption of goodness often is shown to be wrong when studies actually are conducted. Even if the "mean score" is always on the "like" side, individual consumers may not like the product and should have as much opportunity to respond negatively as positively. Also, by destroying balance in the scale, any possibility of having equal intervals in the scale is removed. Clearly, the difference between a 1 assigned "bad" and a 2 assigned to "neither like nor dislike" is a much larger interval (difference) than a 4 assigned to "like moderately" and a 5 assigned to "like very much." Traditional statistical analyses such as t-tests or analysis of variance cannot be used when unbalanced scales are used because those analyses assume that intervals are equal when the scale is converted to numbers.

4. Discrimination and reliability of results often is assumed to increase with an increased number of segments; however, beyond nine points this increase is slight and some researchers have concluded that fewer segments may work as well as more segments. Longer scales do not appear to be warranted except in special cases, which includes scales with many distinct reference points.

5. The number of categories on a scale may be adjusted to the extent of variation likely to be found in the products or qualities evaluated. Keep in mind that for many psychophysical continua (especially taste and aroma characteristics) there are a finite number of perceptual intensity levels (usually fewer than 20) and increasing the number of categories beyond that, even for studies with extreme variation, may not provide additional benefit.

End Anchors for Scales

The words used as end anchors on scales do not appear to create great differentiation with respondents. The use of modifiers such as "extremely" or "very" have not been shown to create problems, nor have they provided the user with "better" data than when no modifier is used. The use of modifiers that are taken from the "popular lingo" have been used with some success, especially with children, but researchers must remember that popular word use changes and modifiers will need to be adjusted if the popular term changes.

Unipolar and Bipolar Scales

Some scales are unipolar and some are bipolar. An example of a unipolar scale would be one to evaluate the intensity of a certain attribute from none to strong.

An example of a bipolar scale would be one to evaluate liking or quality where degrees of both good and bad are meaningful. Whether to use a unipolar or a bipolar scale depends on the characteristic being evaluated. In general, rating scales for intensity should be unipolar because selecting "opposite" words for attributes is difficult. For example, for textile products the opposite of "soft" could be "rough," "stiff," "scratchy," "thick," or many other words. A unipolar measure of each usually is more appropriate.

Special Considerations

In theory the points on rating scales should be equidistant in order to permit statistical analysis by parametric methods. This may be unattainable, in which case the practical objective should be to ensure that the points of the scale are clearly successive and that no successive points are obviously unequal. For example, in a three point scale anchored by "slight," "moderate," and "extreme," the psychological distance from "moderate" to "extreme" may be perceived as larger than from "slight" to "moderate," making "extreme" a poor choice of words on a three-point scale.

Because most scale data are analyzed with statistics by taking a mean value (average), the use of categories that are unequally spaced presents a problem. If the three verbal categories, very slight, slight, and extreme are analyzed by converting them to 1, 2, 3, then the mean of 1 + 2 is 1.5 or 0.5 points lower than slight and the mean of 2 + 3 is 2.5 or 0.5 points higher than slight. But a half point lower than slight is not the same *psychological* distance as a half point higher than slight on this scale. That makes interpretation and subsequent action difficult. Similarly a score of 1 (very slight) and 3 (extreme) would be averaged to 2 (slight), which obviously is not true.

If a verbal scale is to be used, it is important to use simple adverbs and adjectives that are likely to mean the same to most people. The specific words used in completely verbal scales may change the way the scale is used. The use of terms such as "bad," "good," "OK," "poor," "great," "marginal," (all words that have appeared in various scales) is problematic; the words represent a different level of "intensity" of liking to each person. Therefore, the researcher obtains a measure that is as dependent on the perception of the terminology as on the perception of the product. The use of a consistent term such as "dislike" with various modifiers such as "slightly," and "moderately," is preferable.

An important factor bearing on the use of rating scales and, to some degree, on the use of other methods as well, is the dimension of the evaluation specified. It is a frequent fault to specify a quality which may be meaningful to the experimenter, but which the assessors either do not understand or understand in different ways. Care must be taken that each respondent clearly understands the characteristic of each new dimension or attribute specified. Training often is necessary to ensure consistent use of words.

For statistical analysis, successive digits are assigned to the points of the scale, usually beginning at the end representing either zero-intensity or the greatest degree of negative feeling or opinion. This usually follows the convention of having higher numbers represent greater magnitude or more of a given quality or quantity.

In interpreting rating scale data from interval scales it must be remembered that the specific numerical values have no importance, since they have been assigned arbitrarily. However, they certainly can be compared within a test and, with careful planning, may be entered appropriately into a data bank and compared with samples obtained using the same scale with comparable populations.

Magnitude Estimation

This method is similar to the rating scale method in its objectives. Magnitude estimation is, in fact, a special type of rating scale. In magnitude estimation respondents create and employ their own scales rather than those specified by the experimenter. Magnitude estimation generally is less sensitive to "end effects" and "range-frequency" effects than most other rating scales. End effects refer to two phenomena: respondents' avoidance of the extreme categories and the skewing of responses toward one end of the scale. Range-frequency effects refer to the tendency of respondents to try to spread their responses evenly over all available categories.

Magnitude estimation has been applied to a wide range of products and modalities. It has been used for academic research, product development, and consumer research. Magnitude estimation is useful primarily for evaluation of moderate to large suprathreshold differences. The measurement of very small "just noticeable" differences among similar products or sensations is more efficiently accomplished using other sensory techniques. Magnitude estimation also may be useful where a single group of respondents will be used to evaluate and compare a wide range of products and extensive training/orientation for intensities in each product type is not practical.

In magnitude estimation, respondents are instructed to assign numbers to the magnitude of specific sensory attributes using a ratio principle. For example, in estimating odor intensity, respondents would be told that if an odor seemed twice as intense as a previous odor, it should receive a number twice as large. Similarly, if they liked a sample half as much as a previous sample, it should receive a number half as large. Instruction in the method often includes practice exercises in estimating the areas of geometric shapes and the relative pleasantness of a list of words. Emphasis is placed on estimating ratios, using 0 to represent total absence of a particular attribute and the fact that there is no upper limit to the scale.

An identified reference sample or "modulus" sometimes is used to establish a common scale among respondents. When this is done, respondents are given the modulus first and told that it should be assigned a specific value (for example, 13, 24, 2, 50, etc.). Then they assign values to their experimental samples relative to the modulus. The modulus sample may or may not appear as an unidentified sample within the test set. Whether to use a modulus, whether it should reappear within the test set, and what value it should be given must be decided by the investigator on the basis of the nature of the products and attributes being tested. It often is recommended that the intensity of the modulus for the attribute to be studied is close to the geometric mean of the sample set.

When a modulus is not assigned, respondents often are instructed to give their first sample some moderate value (for example, something between 30 and 50). They then evaluate each sample relative to the sample before it.

It generally is agreed that magnitude estimation data are log-normally distributed. It is recommended that all analyses be conducted on data transformed to logarithms. This is not possible for data collected on bipolar scales and presents problems for unipolar data containing zeros because there are no logs of 0's or negative numbers. There are a number of techniques that have been employed for dealing with zeros. These include: replacing all zeros with an arbitrarily small number, replacing zeros with the standard deviation of the data set, adding an arbitrarily small number to each data point, or instructing respondents not to use 0.

When the design and execution of the experiment is appropriate, analysis of variance is the simplest approach to the data analysis. When analysis of variance is not appropriate, it often is necessary to re-scale the data. For example, each respondent's data can be multiplied by a respondent specific factor that brings all the data onto a common scale. One then calculates the geometric mean of the re-scaled data and performs the appropriate statistical tests on the results. NOTE: Much of the literature on magnitude estimation refers to this process as "normalization." However, "normalization" is used in statistics and internationally as a synonym for "standardization." To avoid this conflict, we recommend that the term "re-scaling" be used.

When using magnitude estimation, respondents have a tendency to use "round numbers," that is, 5, 10, 15, 20. This should be noted in training, and respondents should be encouraged to use exact ratios. It has been suggested that the examples used in training can influence the data. Therefore, a variety of different ratios should be used during the training procedures.

Rank Order

The method of rank order can be used to evaluate a set of samples for any attribute that all panel members clearly understand and interpret in the same way. It is more useful when only a short time is needed between samples, as with visual stimuli, than when the time between samples must be extended to minimize the effects of sensory adaptation, as with some odor or taste stimuli.

Usually the ranking task can be done more quickly than evaluation by other methods. Thus, one of the main applications of the method is for rapid preliminary screening in order to identify deviant samples that should be eliminated from further consideration.

For ranking tests, a set of coded samples is presented to each respondent, whose task it is to arrange them in order according to the degree to which they exhibit some specified attribute. Samples also may be arranged according to feelings or opinions about them. All panel members must understand and agree on the criterion on which the samples are to be evaluated. In many cases, such as consumer tests, this requires no more than naming, because there is common understanding of such things as degree of liking, depth of color, intensity of flavor, or even more specific criteria such as the intensity of the fundamental tastes sweet and salty. When an evaluation focuses on characteristics that are less common or pertain to a special product or application, trained respondents, should be employed to assure that common understanding is achieved.

The number of samples in a set may vary from a minimum of three (with only two samples the method becomes paired comparison) to a maximum of about ten. The usual number is four to six samples. The maximum depends upon a number of factors including the sensory modality involved, training and motivation of respondents, the general intensity level of the samples in the set, and the adaptation potential of the material being tested. The permissible limit is greater for trained than for untrained respondents. With untrained respondents no more than four to six samples usually can be included in a set. The number also varies with sense modalities; it is greatest for stimuli that are judged by vision or feeling, next for odor, and least for taste. The method does not work well with chemical feeling factors that linger, such as burn or astringency.

The usual practice is to present all samples of the set at the same time. The respondent is instructed first to examine the samples in succession, following a designated sequence, and establish a preliminary ranking based upon these first impressions. Then the respondent rechecks and verifies this order, making any changes that seem to be warranted. Samples may be presented monadically (singularly in succession), so that the experimenter has full control over the sequence of examination. However, monadic presentation detracts from a main advantage of the method, that is, ease of administration. Also, a respondent cannot recheck the preliminary ranking or make direct, quick comparison if samples are presented monadically.

The order of sample presentation in the first trial is important because of potential sensory adaptation and contrast effects. Order may have little or no effect with visual or tactile dimensions, because samples can be evaluated with little time lag between them and adaptation may be only a minor concern; however, with taste and odor stimuli and sometimes with color stimuli, the phenomena of adaptation and recovery must be considered. The order usually is controlled by the way the samples are presented and instructions to the respondents, for example, try the samples in order from left to right. The order should be balanced as much as possible within the limitations of panel size, so that each sample is tried in each position of the sequence about equally often. After the initial ranking has been completed, there usually is no restriction placed on the sequence of rechecking the samples.

When dealing with samples where sensory adaptation is important, special precautions must be made. During the first examination of the set, and during subsequent rechecking, a suitable interval must be allowed between samples. The length of the interval may vary with the nature of the material being evaluated, principally the intensity and persistence of the stimulus. Whether the nature of the samples will allow less time or require a greater interval is a matter for the experimenter's judgment, aided by the respondents' observations. When all samples are presented at the same time, the interval between samples must be estimated or timed by the respondents. To do this accurately may require special training, instructions, or use of equipment such as timers or a metronome. When left to their own devices, most people will over-estimate how much time has passed and will not allow long enough intervals, or the intervals may vary in length.

Special Considerations on Data Analysis for Rank Order Tests

One way to present rank order results is in terms of the average rank for each sample, which is the sum of all of the individual rankings divided by the number of rankings. Of course, these averages are meaningless outside the context of a particular experiment.

The recommended method of analysis of rank order data is Friedman's test, which is a special application of chi-square. The analysis first determines whether or not the overall distribution of the rank totals for a set of samples is significantly different from that expected by chance. If so, then an extension of the analysis may be used to calculate the least significant difference (LSD), which is the amount of difference between rank totals which may be considered as significant (see Chapter 7 on Statistics).

A procedure that sometimes is used is to treat the rankings as if they were rating scale data. The results closely approximate those obtained by Friedman's analysis; however, the procedure violates certain statistical assumptions.

Formerly, a procedure based upon Kramer's table of rank sums often was employed to analyze rank order data. However, early tables were found to contain errors. The method can be used if the more recent, corrected tables are available, and with the understanding that comparisons of intermediate ranked samples should be made only to samples of the highest or lowest rank, not to other intermediate ranked samples.

Ranking: Case Study

Objective

Determine the most appropriate shapes for components of a pet food product.

Test Method

Ranking tests were selected for this study because degree of liking was not important to the decision-making process and further testing was planned after several product options were determined. These tests also were selected for efficiency because one group of respondents could easily do four sets of visual rankings in one session. Ranks were, assigned from 1: most appropriate to 3: least appropriate. This test was repeated for the shape of each product component, but only one component (beef and chicken) is reported here.

Results

Data for Ranking for Pet Food Component Shapes			
Respondent	Drumstick	Figure 8	Small Nugget
1	1	2	3
2	1	2	3
3	1	2	3
4	2	1	3
5	2	3	1
6	3	1	2
7	1	2	3
8	1	2	3
9	1	2	3
10	2	1	3
11	2	3	1
12	3	2	1
13	1	2	3
14	1	2	3
15	1	3	2
16	1	2	3
17	1	3	2
18	2	3	1
19	2	1	3
20	1	3	2
21	1	2	3
22	1	3	2
Total Sums	32	47	53

The test statistic used to determine if there are differences in the rank sums of the samples is

$$T = [(12/bt(t + 1)) \, \Sigma R_i^2] - 3b(t + 1)$$

where

$b =$ number of respondents,
$t =$ number of samples, and
$R_i =$ rank sum for sample i.

For this example

$$T = [(12/(22)(3)(3 + 1))(32^2 + 47^2 + 53^2)] - 3(22)(3 + 1)$$
$$= [(1/22)(6042)] - 264$$
$$= 10.64$$

The test statistic follows a chi-square distribution with $t - 1$ degrees of freedom. Based on the critical values of the chi-square distribution with two degrees of freedom in Chapter 7 Table 5, it is seen that $T = 10.64$ exceeds the $\alpha = 0.05$ critical significantly in appropriateness. To determine which shapes are significantly different an LSD (least significant difference) value was calculated using

$$\text{LSD} = \frac{z_\alpha}{2\sqrt{\dfrac{bt(t + 1)}{6}}} = 1.96\sqrt{\frac{22 \cdot 3 \cdot 4}{6}} = 13$$

Any two rank sums that differ by more than the LSD value are significantly different. Therefore, the "drumstick" was found to be a significantly more appropriate shape for the beef and chicken component than either the "Figure 8" or the "Small Nugget." There was no significant difference between the "Figure 8" and the "Small Nugget" shapes.

Recommendation

Based on these data, it is recommended that acceptance tests now be conducted to determine the liking of the product with all four components. Two test products with various shapes for the components were recommended for the follow-up test.

Just-About-Right Scaling Method

The just-about-right (JAR) rating scale, commonly is used in marketing research to identify product attributes that may require improvement. Naive respondents (consumers) indicate whether a product is about right for a specified product attribute or if there is too much or too little of that attribute. It is a bimodal scale, adapted from use in the study of social issues and attitudes about people and events.

The scale usually is intended to be used with a panel size of 100 or more. It is assumed that the naive respondent will understand the attributes, as well as how to use the scale. The scale often is used as a three point scale, and when it is longer, it often is condensed by researchers to three points for ease of analysis. This scale usually is insensitive to small differences and there are other scaling methods and analyses that often are better suited to sensory evaluation. However, it does have limited use in screening and product guidance.

In JAR scaling the consumer is requested to indicate whether the product is about right or if not; is it too weak or too strong; too little or too much; too light or too dark; or other "opposite" terms. Typically the scale is used as part of a test in which other product questions are asked, for example, degree of liking. The scale is verbally anchored with just-about-right in the center and equal numbers of categories on both sides; for example, too weak and too strong. An example with five-points is:

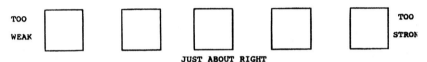

The scale is not a continuum but a series of discrete categories. There can be as many as four categories on each side, but the larger the number of categories the more likely the terminology will be confusing; for example, a color scale with three categories on each side—light, too light, and much too light or dark, too dark, and much too dark. Consumers easily can be confused as to the difference between light and too light, and whether one is measuring intensities or qualities. In other cases using more than one category on each side of just about-right can be cumbersome as well as confusing. For example, "slightly too spicy" and "much too spicy" make sense, as does "not spicy enough." However, trying to measure degrees of "not spicy enough" can be difficult to understand.

Attention must be given to how the method will be used and specifically how the results will be analyzed. Because the JAR scale is a dichotomous scale, the suggested analyses are limited to percentage of judgments in the center and on each side (low and high), or the serial use of a chi-square methodology; the Stuart-Maxwell and the McNemar tests are typical (for information on chi-square see Chapter 7 on Statistics). The percentage of judgments in a category is the most commonly used approach. Some companies use standard percentages such as a minimum 70% of responses in the just-about-right category to determine if a product attribute is considered to be acceptable. If that criteria is met then nothing further is done. If the percentage is less than the standard level, it is assumed that product change is warranted in the direction, higher or lower, that has the greater percentage of respondents.

Just About Right Scale: Case Study

Objective

To determine if the levels of two attributes (sweetness, crunchiness) are more appropriate in Product A or Product B (the competitor) and to give direction for changing the intensities in product A if they are not "JUST RIGHT".

Test Method

The just about right scale was selected in order to get a "quick read" on differences in the acceptability of the intensities of two attributes. A 3 category just-about-right scale was used and data were collected from 100 respondents.

Results

Responses for Level of Sweetness	N	Too Sweet	About Right	Not Sweet Enough
Product A	100	3 (3%)	81 (81%)	17 (17%)
Product B	100	11 (11%)	64 (64%)	25 (25%)

Responses for Crunchiness	N	Too Crunchy	About Right	Not Crunchy Enough
Product A	100	42 (42%)	47 (47%)	11 (11%)
Product B	100	3 (3%)	86 (86%)	11 (11%)

Findings

The data indicated that the sweetness of Product A may be perceived ás more appropriate than the level in B by a larger percentage of the respondents. The data for crunchiness indicated that the crunchiness of Product A was much less appropriate than for Product B, and suggested that Product A probably is too crunchy for most consumers.

Recommendation

Based on these sensory data, it was recommended that further development be conducted to reduce the perceived crunchiness of Product A without affecting sweetness.

Bibliography

Anderson, N. H., "Algebraic Rules in Psychological Measurement," *American Scientist,* Vol. 67, Sept.–Oct. 1979, pp. 555–563.

Alexander, H. H., Alexander, M. A., and Tzeng, O. C. S., "Designing Semantic Differential Scales for a Universe of the Near Environment—Chairs," *Home Economics Research Journal,* Vol. 6, No. 4, 1978, pp. 293–304.

Chapman, L. D. and Wigfield, R., "Rating Scales in Consumer Research," *Food Manufacture*, Aug. 1970, pp. 59–62.

Giovànni, M. E. and Pangborn, R. M., "Measurement of Taste Intensity and Degree of Liking of Beverages by Graphic Scales and Magnitude Estimation," *Journal of Food Science*, Vol. 48, No. 4, 1983, pp. 1175–1182.

Kroll, B. J., "Evaluating Rating Scales for Sensory Testing with Children," *Food Technology*, Vol. 44, No. 11, Nov. 1990, pp. 78–80, 82, 84, 86.

Land, D. G. and Shepherd, R.,"Scaling and Ranking Methods," *Sensory Analysis of Foods*, J. R. Piggott, Ed., Elsevier, New York, 1984, pp. 141–177.

Lawless, H. T. and Malone, G. J., "The Discriminative Efficiency of Common Scaling Methods," *Journal of Sensory Studies*, Vol. 1, No. 1, 1986, pp. 85–98.

Lawless, H. T. and Malone, G. J., "Comparison of Rating Scales: Sensitivity, Replicates, and Relative Measurement," *Journal of Sensory Studies*, Vol. 1, No. 2, 1986, pp. 151–174.

McDaniel, M. R. and Sawyer, F. M., "Descriptive Analysis of Whiskey Sour Formulations: Magnitude Estimation Versus a 9-Point Category Scale," *Journal of Food Science*, Vol. 46, 1981, pp. 178–189.

Moskowitz, H. R. and Sidel, J. L., "Magnitude and Hedonic Scales of Food Acceptability," *Journal of Food Science*, Vol. 36, 1971, pp. 677–680.

Moskowitz, H. R., "Applications of Sensory Measurement to Food Evaluation. II. Methods of Ratio Scaling," *Lebensmittel-Wisseascharf und Technologie*, Vol. 9, 1976, pp. 249–254.

Moskowitz, H. R., "Respondent and Response Types in Magnitude Estimation Scaling," *Food Product and Development*, Vol. 11, No. 5, May 1977, pp. 95–98.

Orth, B. and Wegener, B., "Scaling Occupational Prestige by Magnitude Estimation and Category Rating Methods: A Comparison with the Sensory Domain," *European Journal of Social Psychology*, Vol. 13, 1983, pp. 417–431.

Pearce, J. H., Korth, B., and Warren, C. B., "Evaluation of Three Scaling Methods for Hedonics," *Journal of Sensory Studies, Sensory Analysis of Foods*, Vol. 1, No. 1, pp. 27–46.

Peryam, D. R. and Pilgrim, F. J., "Hedonic Scale Method of Measuring Food Preferences," *Food Technology*, Vol. 11, No. 9, 1957, pp. 9–14.

Schmidt, D. J. and Hoff, J. T., "Use of Graphic Linear Scales to Measure Rates of Staling in Beer," *Journal of Food Science*, Vol. 44, 1979, pp. 901–904.

Shand, P. J., Hawrysh, Z. J., Hardin, R. T., and Jeremiah, L. E., "Descriptive Sensory Assessment of Beef Steaks by Category Scaling, Line Scaling and Magnitude Estimation," *Journal of Food Science*, Vol. 50, No. 2, 1985, pp. 495–500.

Spaeth, E. E., Chambers, E. IV, and Schwenke, J. R., "A Comparison of Acceptability Scaling Methods for Use with Children," *Product Testing with Consumers for Research Guidance: Special Consumer Groups, ASTM STP 1155*, L. S. Wu and A. D. Gelinas, Eds., American Society for Testing and Materials, Philadelpia, 1992, pp. 65–77.

Stevens, S. S. and Galanter, E. H., "Ratio Scales and Category Scales for a Dozen Perceptual Continua," *Journal of Experimental Psychology*, Vol. 54, No. 6, 1957, pp. 377–411.

Stevens, S. S., "The Surprising Simplicity of Sensory Metrics," *American Psychology*, Vol. 17, pp. 29–39.

Chapter 4—Threshold Methods

Threshold methods are designed for the specific purposes of determining the strength or concentration of a stimulus required to produce: a minimal detectable effect (detection threshold), recognizable effect (recognition threshold), or change in effect (difference threshold). In any threshold method there can be two criteria for response: one is detection, in which the respondent has only to respond to differences from some product or background, and the other is recognition, in which the respondent must name the specific stimulus, for example, "salt" or "strong."

Threshold methods are labor-intensive and time consuming, and the quantity measured, "the lowest intensity a person can detect," is vague and elusive; it is affected by chance variations in mood and in physical conditions; it is surprisingly variable from moment to moment and from day to day, and it is highly variable between individual respondents. No definite value is obtained but rather a series of judgments which require sophisticated statistical treatment to produce a value and confidence limits. A single threshold determination can take a week and yet be off by an order of magnitude, so that many repeats are needed to establish a reliable value. Threshold methods are an analyst's tool of last resort, but there are situations where no other method will serve.

Typically thresholds are determined "for an added substance," that is, for a compound or a product added to a neutral reference medium. Detection thresholds in odorless air are used to determine degrees of air pollution and to set legal limits for polluters. Thresholds of added pure substances are used with water supplies, foods, beverages, cosmetics, paints, solvents, textiles, etc. to determine the point at which known contaminants begin to affect acceptability. These are the most important uses, and tests may be done with hundreds of respondents in order to map the relative sensitivities of the population. The threshold of added desirable substances may be used as a research tool in the formulation of paints, fragrances, foods, beverages, etc. Effects of difference threshold also may be determined for an ingredient or a process variation in a product. To make the results of a threshold test applicable to general use, the sensory purity of the added substance, as well as the purity of the neutral reference medium, should be as high as possible, or it should be typical of the component. Purity data should be recorded together with the threshold. It is likely that many threshold data in the literature are artificially low because of the presence of highly-flavored impurities in the stimulus used. In test series of pure chemicals, detection thresholds for certain compounds (mercaptans, pyrazines, and other heterocycles) can be lower by a factor of up to 10^{12} compared with simple compounds (alcohols, lipids, carbohydrates); hence, chemical purity, even 99.99%, is no guarantee of sensory purity. Thresholds reported in the literature often differ by several orders of magnitude.

The method by which the stimulus is presented must be specified, as it can strongly affect the threshold. For example, in odor threshold tests, an odorant flow of 100 mL/s produced thresholds several-fold lower than a flow of 1 to 2 L/s. The use of a larger sniff bottle resulted in 10 to 20-fold lower thresholds. Training raises the ability to recognize and detect the stimulus, often by 100-fold in the case of lesser-known odors or tastes. Despite these limitations, researchers may find published data useful in establishing rough approximations of stimulus levels required to produce an effect. However, use of published data, for example, as air quality criteria is not recommended; for this, a test should be done under conditions simulating actual exposure and using respondents from the population exposed.

Thresholds may be determined: (*a*) for a single respondent or (*b*) for a group. Experience shows that individual thresholds can vary 2- to 4-fold or occasionally 10-fold from one test to another. Variations between individuals are much larger and can reach 1000-fold or more. Not infrequently, a respondent is found to vary even more from the norm, that is, showing partial or even full anosmia or ageusia for a particular stimulus, and deviating by a million-fold or more. ASTM takes the position [E 1432-91] that determination of the threshold for a group is a two-step process that must begin with a determination of the individual thresholds. The frequency distribution of these is examined and depending on its form, the group threshold is chosen as that measure of central tendency best suited to the data; for example the median, the average, the mode, or the geometric mean; or, it may be found that the group consists of one or more subgroups, each with a different group threshold. A simplified example of calculation is found in Chapter 7. The remainder of the present chapter deals with individual thresholds only. For more detail, see the following publications: E 1432-91 for a detailed method and E 679-91 for abbreviated method, suitable for a rough evaluation of a group.

Preparation of Samples

In a typical determination of the threshold of an individual respondent, a series of samples is prepared representing increasing concentrations of the stimulus of interest in the selected diluent. The series is such that it brackets the range in which the threshold lies with six to ten steps. Use of a log series of concentrations (that is, with fixed ratios of two or more) is recommended. Preliminary examination and testing is required to locate the appropriate range. For a detection threshold, the lowest step of the range is located at a near-zero concentration. For difference or recognition thresholds, the range may start at a point definitely higher than the standard. The use of blanks (no stimulus) within a test series is recommended in order to reduce response bias and the effects of guessing on the result.

Selected Methods

Three test paradigms (test philosophies and resulting setups) are in common use for determination of thresholds (see Kling & Riggs, 1971): the Method of

Constant Stimuli, the Method of Limits, and Dilution Techniques. (Different models of the threshold, derived from Decision Analysis and Signal Detection Theory, are also in use but not included here). Each method can be applied to all three types of threshold, detection, recognition, and difference; for recognition the detection criterion becomes "the concentration at which the stimulus is correctly identified" and the respondent is trained what to look for.

The Method of Constant Stimuli

Each sample is paired with the standard or reference; for detection thresholds the standard is zero concentration. The pairs are presented in random order. The respondent judges which sample in each pair is stronger. That point in the series at which 50% of the judgments are correct is designated the threshold. "Correct" means "agrees with the direction of the stimulus concentration difference." Often, to reduce the effects of response bias, the paired comparison is replaced by the 3-alternative forced choice (3-AFC) test, in which the respondent knows that one of three samples contains the stimulus, the other two do not; the respondent must choose which sample contains the stronger stimulus. The concentration corresponding to 50% correct judgment, adjusted for guessing, is recorded as the threshold. Response bias is a problem if a respondent lacks motivation to discriminate or conversely, if a respondent records a difference where none is perceived in order to appear more discriminating.

The Method of Limits

The samples are presented in order of physical concentration, and the respondents judge the presence or absence of the designated quality. Often, ascending series (starting with a below-threshold stimulus) and descending series are given alternately. A series is continued until the judgment changes (from yes to no, or vice versa) and stays the same for two successive presentations. Blanks (zero concentrations) may be used in the series. A single threshold is the average of the values obtained in an ascending and a descending series.

ASTM Methods E 679-91 and E 1432-91 are based on a variation of this method in which samples are presented only in an ascending series of stimulus concentrations in order to reduce the effects of carry-over and fatigue. A forced-choice method of presentation is used, and the concentration at which the proportion of correct responses is 50% above chance is recorded as the threshold.

Dilution Techniques

Dilution methods represent an application of threshold measurement techniques to practical situations, in which the problem is to obtain a measure of the difference between test products and a standard, when the difference is a complex result of the processing received by the product. The methods may vary with regard to certain particulars but are basically the same; they have been used, for example, with dried whole milk, with dried eggs, and with perfumes and other products. Dilution is often used for air quality tests.

A dilution threshold test begins with the selection of an appropriate standard product. Next, an upper limit for the series is established, that is, the highest concentration or change in process which it is reasonable to subject to formal testing. This has to be done by trial and error, but it is often sufficient to ask two or three people, who are known discriminators for the stimulus in question, to indicate the lowest change in process that definitely will be perceptible.

1. In similar fashion, select a lower limit (above zero) for the series such that it is very unlikely that any respondent will be able to reliably detect a difference between it and the standard.

2. Define a series of process steps including the upper and lower limits just defined. Usually six steps are enough, although eight may be used if greater precision is desired. Space the steps at equal sensory intervals; often this means a log concentration scale.

Present each step in the series to the panel together with the reference and determine the weakest step which is perceived as different. Again the threshold is that step for which the proportion of "different" verdicts is 50% above chance. If needed, reduce response bias by presenting the samples as 3-AFC or duo-trio tests (at the expense of sensory fatigue which in turn limits the number of process variations that can be tested).

The threshold obtained by this technique is a measure of the degree of difference between the test method of production and the standard. The selection of the reference standard is a matter of judgment. It must be meaningful in relation to the product and the problem represented.

Often, an isolated result has little practical value, and the method is appropriate only when there is a need for evaluation and comparing a number of treatments of the same product type. This has implications for the selection of the reference standard: it must be a material whose flavor will not change from one source of supply to another.

Bibliography

Amoore, J. E. and Hautala, E., "Odor as an Aid to Chemical Safty: Odor Thresholds Compared with Threshold Limit Values and Volatilities for 214 Industrial Chemicals in Air and Water Dilution," *Journal of Applied Toxicology,* Vol. 3, No. 6, 1993, pp. 272–290.

ASTM, 1991, E 1432-91, *Standard Practice for Defining and Calculating Individual and Group Sensory Thresholds from Forced-Choice Data Sets of Intermediate Size,* ASTM Volume 15.07, American Society for Testing and Materials, Philadelphia.

ASTM, 1991, E 679-91, *Standard Practice for Determination of Odor and Taste Thresholds by a Forced-Choice Ascending Concentration Series Method of Limits,* ASTM Volume 15.07, American Society for Testing and Materials, Philadelphia.

Kling, J. W. and Riggs, L. A., *Woodworth & Schlosberg's Experimental Psychology, 3rd Edition,* Chapter 2. Holt, Rinehart & Winston, New York, 1971.

Stahl, W. H., *Compilation of Odor and Taste Threshold Values Data,* American Society for Testing and Materials, Philadelphia, 1973.

Chapter 5—Descriptive Analysis

Descriptive analysis is one of the most common forms of sensory testing. Descriptive methods are used to measure the type and intensity of attributes in a product. Thus, these methods require the respondent to describe a product in terms of its characteristics and to measure the intensity of those characteristics using scaling procedures. Although some attributes are fairly simple and can be measured easily by almost anyone, real understanding of a product's specific characteristics and the strength of the attributes requires the use of respondents trained to describe sensory stimuli and to measure intensity of perception.

Descriptive sensory information is used in a variety of ways. It may serve to "fingerprint" a product for later comparison to new batches or other products. Control charts can be developed and maintained for critical sensory characteristics that are measured for quality assurance. Descriptive information may be compared among a variety of products to determine the differences that currently are available in the marketplace. Using various statistical techniques, researchers can attempt to relate these data to consumer acceptance, physical, or chemical measurements. In some instances, descriptive characteristics of products are used to develop advertising campaigns that stress a product's unique properties or emphasize those characteristics that are the product's strength. Numerous other uses of descriptive information can be found and other uses are sure to develop.

The use of language is very important in descriptive analysis. One must be concerned not only with what is perceived but also with how the information is transmitted by the respondent. This can become a major source of variability in the test results. The "assumption of same word-one meaning" often is made but sometimes may not be true. The researcher should be aware of the possibility of semantic error and attempt to reduce it. Devices commonly employed to eliminate, or reduce, the error arising from this source include the use of definitions agreed on by the respondents, physical reference standards, and intensive training of respondents.

Several descriptive sensory "systems" have been published, the main ones being Flavor Profile, Texture Profile, Quantitative Descriptive Analysis (QDA), and Spectrum Analysis. Many variations of those methods are used and scientists tailor the techniques to fit their unique situation. One issue of special importance is that the selection and training of respondents is not easy; it is time consuming and requires some special skills. Anyone who wants to develop a trained panel should seek the assistance of sensory experts experienced in the descriptive methods.

Flavor Profile Method

The Flavor Profile is a method describing the aroma and flavor of products or ingredients. It is based on the concept that flavor consists of identifiable taste, odor, and chemical feeling attributes, plus an underlying complex of attributes not separately identifiable.

The method consists of formal procedures for describing and assessing the flavor of a product in a reproducible manner. The separate attributes contributing to the overall sensory impression/amplitude of the product are identified and their intensity assessed in order to build a description of the flavor of the product.

A descriptive analysis of flavor usually includes: (1) overall impression of aroma and flavor (amplitude), (2) identification of perceptible aroma and flavor notes, (3) degree of intensity of each aroma and flavor note, (4) order in which the notes are perceived (order of appearance), and (5) identification of aftertaste.

The members of a Flavor Profile Panel are selected and trained by experts in the method. Respondents are selected on the basis of a series of screening tests that include fundamental tastes, odor recognition, taste intensity recognition, taste intensity ranking, and a personal interview to evaluate availability and personality traits. Training is done over a period of six to twelve months. It includes fundamental sensory principles and training in all aspects of the Flavor Profile technique. At the conclusion of training, a permanent panel leader (or leaders) is chosen.

After completion of training, four to eight respondents work as a group to arrive at a description of the flavor of a product. The panel leader leads the discussion to reach a consensus on each component of the profile. Reference materials and more than one panel session usually are required in order to reach the consensus. The panel leader interprets and reports the results. An orientation period of one or more sessions often is helpful. The samples to be studied are introduced, and similar products may be brought in for comparison. A list of the flavor notes is compiled, reference samples decided upon, and the best methods of presentation and examining of samples established.

Formal panel sessions follow, in which each panel member independently evaluates the samples and records his or her findings. Aroma and flavor notes and feeling factors, their intensities, their order of appearance, and aftertaste are recorded. The intensity scale is used as follows:

) (= threshold (barely perceptible)
1 = slight
2 = moderate
3 = strong

The intensity scale often is further divided into 1/2 units or + and − units.

The overall impression, or amplitude, is a general assessment of the product-considering the unidentifiable background flavor, the blend of flavors, the appropriateness of aroma and flavor notes present, and their intensities, the amplitude rating scale is 3 (high), 2 (medium), and (1) low, and it also may be refined into 1/2 units.

Individual results are compiled by the panel leader. An open discussion follows and disagreements are discussed until a consensus is reached. Multiple panel sessions usually are necessary. A final profile is then composed by the panel leader. Results are often presented as a vertical, tabular profile; however, they may also be presented graphically. The panel leader reports the results in a manner that is meaningful to those who are familiar or unfamiliar with the Flavor Profile method. A report usually consists of the tabular profile as well as a discussion of the profile in paragraph form.

Flavor Profile Method: Case Study

Objective

To understand the strengths and weaknesses of the flavor of four major brands of liquid antacids in order to more easily and effectively design a new product entry into the antacid category.

Test Method

Using five trained and experienced flavor profile respondents, the information presented in Fig. 1 was obtained within one week. A total of six 30 min. panel sessions was held with two products evaluated at each session. Findings from the analysis of the first product were compiled prior to analysis of the second product, thus providing time for recovery of taste buds and avoiding carry-over of sensory effect.

Two products were presented coded, in 50-mL beakers to the five respondents at each of the six panel sessions. As soon as the respondents were assembled and ready to start, each respondent took about 2/3 teaspoon of the liquid, swallowed it, and started to write down the aromatic, taste, and mouth feel sensations. This was repeated until a total dose of 2 teaspoons (and no more) had been tested, and as much information as possible recorded. After data from the second analysis of each individual product were compiled, the respondents were presented with a fairly detailed profile for their third analysis. Final flavor profiles resulted from the changes and additions at the third panel session.

Using the final Flavor Profiles, the panel leader then started the interpretation of the data. A report summarizing the data, conclusions, and recommendations was prepared for subsequent action.

Results

Some significant facts were immediately apparent, as each product demonstrated a discernible difference from the other three. Product A had the most paraben effects (refers to the *p*-aminobenzoic acid compounds used as antimicrobial), including a definite gauze-like aromatic with numbing and tongue and throat sting. The dominance of these factors can be attributed to the type of paraben used, concentration used, and possibly the source of the compound, as well as to the lack of coverage provided by the minty flavor and cooling mouth

Product A (Amplitude 1)		Product B (Amplitude 1½)		Product C (Amplitude ½)		Product D (Amplitude 1)	
Flavor-by-mouth							
Sweet	1½	Sweet		Sweet	1→1½	Sweet	2
Cooling	1½	Lemony (terpy,waxy)	1½→2	Minty (old)/menthol	1½	Vanilla, vanillin	½
Minty	1	Medicinal, parabens	1→1½	Medicinal (parabens)	1½	Minty, (spt, ppf)	1
Parabens (gauze)	1½→2	Chalky MF	2	Chalky MF	1	Cooling	2
Chalky MF	1½	Astringent	1½	Cooling	1½→2	Parabens (gauze)	2
Drying	1½	Drying	1	SSS	1	Bitter	1
Numbing, tongue sting	2	Numbing	1	Bitter	1	Tongue sting/numbing	½
Aftertaste (1 min. after swallow)							
Chalky MF	1	Chalky MF	1½	Cooling	1	Cooling	1
Parabens, numbing & sting	1	Throat burn	1½	Drying	1	Chalky MF	1
Throat sting	1	Mouth sting	1	Bitter	1	Parabens & sting	1
Bitter	1	Drying	1	SSS	1	Throat burn	½
Sour	1						
Cooling	1						
Viscosity							
V. sl. thick (like cream)		Watery		Watery		Sl. thick (maple syrup)	
Texture							
V. sl. gritty; feels smooth		Chalky		Chalky, sl. gritty		Smooth	

FIG. 1—Flavor profiles of OTC antacids 2 teaspoon dose (10 mL)

feel. Product D on the other hand had the most cooling and a more complex flavoring system (vanilla and minty). These factors provided some, although not enough, diversion from the paraben effects as their intensities were about as strong as in Product A.

Product B had the highest amplitude of the group, probably due to the more intense flavoring which appeared to blend the other sensory impressions. The paraben effect was lower than in Products A and D. However, the chalky mouth feel was more noticeable and the flavoring did not last into the aftertaste to provide coverage of the chalkiness, mouth burn, and sting.

Product C was unique in that it had a noticeable saccharin effect described as SSS (synthetic sweetener sensation). Additionally, the minty flavor was described as old (dried leaves) and did not have the intensity or bouquet to cover the medicinal paraben effect, or to last into the aftertaste.

A review of all the profiles indicated two major flavor problems probably inherent in the product category: chalky mouth feel and the paraben effect. However, there were differences in the ways these were manifested which suggests that it is possible to deal with these constraints.

Recommendations

The important points to incorporate in the product development/improvement effort are that the new product should have: a complex flavoring system including some citrus, some brown flavor (vanillin, vanilla) and some minty notes that will last into aftertaste; a combination of different parabens to result in the least flavor contribution; possible use of a nutritive sweetener.

Texture Profile

The texture profile method was developed to focus on aspects that were overlooked in the flavor profile. Texture profile assumes, as do all descriptive methods, that texture is made up of many attributes and that the intensity and order of the attributes can be measured. The original procedure for texture profiling has been modified to provide for more precision, new attributes and scaling procedures, use of individual scores instead of consensus (where warranted), statistical analysis, and products other than food.

The principle of texture profile is that attributes of texture can be divided into three categories: mechanical, geometrical, and other characteristics (primarily fat and moisture). The attributes are defined and measured using a numerical scale of standards developed for each attribute. The standards, generally commercially available products, have been established and published and are widely used. Modifications of the scales are used and developed when certain standards are not available, have changed, or when finer gradations are needed in the scale.

Respondents are selected using many of the criteria for other sensory descriptive studies. Because the work focuses on texture, a special emphasis on issues such as dental health or manual dexterity often is placed on selecting respondents for this and other methods that require products to be chewed.

Generally, texture profiling follows procedures common among descriptive methods for texture, and determining and defining attributes. Perhaps more than any other method, an emphasis is placed on referencing each specific scale with a number of examples that are specific to that attribute.

The panel works under a panel leader, who is a sensory professional, and is responsible for the operation of the panel, analysis of data, and interpretation and reporting of results. The individual also is a trained texture profile respondent, but rarely sits on a panel because of biases related to knowledge of the test.

Orientation sessions are held and respondents can review commercial products and test prototypes. Specific attention is paid to standardizing the way the product is manipulated. For example, how food is manipulated in the mouth, how it is bitten, how many chews, the rate of chewing, and when to swallow.

Texture profiling typically has been conducted in a test facility that encourages discussion, but increasingly is being conducted in individual booths without a requirement that consensus be reached. Data are compiled into tabular form and reported along with an interpretive statement, if necessary, similar to the flavor profile.

Quantitative Descriptive Analysis

The quantitative descriptive analysis (QDA) method is a type of trained panel procedure in which all the sensory properties of a product are described and their intensities quantified. The QDA method uses ten to twelve qualified respondents who are users/acceptors of the products being tested and have demonstrated they can discriminate differences among the products being tested. In a typical situation, about 60% of those who volunteer will meet this sensory skill requirement.

The respondents, working under direction of the panel leader, develop a sensory language, or modify an existing one, to describe all of the products' sensory properties. The respondents group the attributes by modality (aroma, appearance, etc.), order them within a modality, and develop definitions for each one of them. The subjects also develop a standardized evaluation procedure. A final task is to practice scoring the products. There are no limits as to the number of attributes that the panel develops, only that they agree as to their names and their order on the scorecard. These training activities require from 6 to 10 h, usually organized into 90-min sessions. The panel leader's primary responsibilities are to organize the training, provide the products, introduce references when needed, and facilitate the activities, but not to function as a respondent.

At the conclusion of training, the panel evaluates all the products using a repeated trials design. For most tests, a four replicate design is sufficient to provide for analysis.

The analysis provides measures of respondent performance on an attribute basis, the usefulness of each attribute in differentiating products, and product differences, also on an attribute basis. The analysis of variance (see Chapter 7 on Statistics), using a mixed model, and least squares solution is the primary methodology; however, there are numerous other parametric and nonparametric analyses done to verify the quality of the database, the integrity of the statistical conclusions, and verification of the conclusions reached. Results can be presented in a numerical format or in a graphical representation. The methodology is used for all types of products, including foods, beverages, personal care, home care, fabrics, and so forth.

QDA Method: Case Study

Objectives

1. Determine effect of a new processing method on the flavor and texture of crackers by comparing attributes of stamped crackers (standard method) versus rotary cut crackers and

2. Determine whether added salt spray (2%) increased wheat flavor perception of the rotary cut (test) product.

Methods

The QDA procedure was selected because many different characteristics of aroma, appearance, flavor, and texture needed to be studied. Twelve trained respondents from the cracker QDA panel were used. Each respondent received all three products on each of three days in a Latin square design that balanced order of presentation. The serving size was four crackers served in a cup with a sealed lid. Six aroma attributes, six appearance attributes, seven flavor attributes, five aftertaste attributes, and five texture attributes were evaluated on each sample. The scale was a 6 in. (12.7 cm) line scale anchored 0.5 in. (1.27 cm) from each end with either none or extreme. Respondents marked the line for intensity of each attribute and the intensities were read to the nearest tenth of an inch using a digitizing pad. Data were analyzed using analysis of variance.

Results

Data are given only for one attribute in this case study (overall flavor impact), but would be given for each attribute when reported.

	Overall flavor impact	
	Without Salt	With Salt
Stamped	3.5	not tested
Rotary Cut	4.4	5.1

The rotary cut cracker, with salt spray, had more overall flavor impact (probably caused by the salt) and much more saltiness (observed in flavor, and aftertaste) than either of the unsalted products. Both rotary cut products had slightly more overall flavor impact than the standard.

Conclusions

The rotary cut product was similar in flavor and texture to the standard cracker. Some appearance and flavor differences were apparent and need to be investigated further. Salt appeared to add saltiness and overall flavor, but did not change other characteristics.

Spectrum Descriptive Analysis Method

In the Spectrum method the perceived intensities are recorded in relation to absolute, or universal scales, that are constant for all products and attributes. A Spectrum panel is trained in a variety of attribute modalities or as an alternative, it can emphasize any one of the sensory modalities to fit the project needs. This method is used to evaluate an array of product categories, including foods, beverages, personal care, home care, paper, and other products.

Respondents are selected based on six major criteria: perceptual ability, rating ability, interest, availability, attitudes to task and products, and health. For the final selection of 15 respondents (10 to 12 who will be used on any particular project), approximately 60 to 80 people are recruited to participate in the pre-screening. This number provides a sufficiently large pool for obtaining qualified respondents through the two stages of screening. Acuity tests are dependent on the type of training to be conducted (for example, flavor, texture, skin feel). The tests are designed to select respondents who are discriminators of the sensory characteristics to be evaluated.

The training is completed in two phases: orientation and practice phases. The orientation sessions cover the physiological principles for the sensory modalities of interest and procedures used to evaluate them. During practice sessions, demonstrations are conducted that allow the respondents to practice and apply the principles learned during the orientation sessions. A total of 10 to 12 exercises are conducted during the three or more months of panel work, needed to understand the modalities of interest. Three major tasks are completed for each exercise: (1) review of samples representing the product category and preliminary terminology development, (2) review of product references and establishment of terminology and evaluation procedures, and (3) product evaluation and discussion of results. The panel is ready for formal evaluation after this time and after its performance has been assessed by the trainer and panel leader.

One or several orientation sessions are conducted prior to the product evaluation sessions. To establish the attributes (ballot) and evaluation procedures needed to fully characterize the test products, actual test products, commercial products and an extensive array of qualitative and quantitative references are presented in the session(s).

Each respondent individually evaluates the test products following the established ballot and evaluation procedures. The evaluation is usually conducted in duplicate or triplicate in separate evaluation sessions. Data are collected and analyzed statistically. The statistical analysis used depends on the project objective and the experimental design. At the end of a series of evaluations or projects the panel and panel leader are encouraged to meet to discuss problems and references used during the study. This type of discussion after completion of a study is valuable for improving panel evaluation, performance, and to resolve problems.

The Spectrum descriptive analysis method provides: (1) a description of the major product sensory categories, (2) a detailed separation and description of each sensory attribute within each major sensory category and with specific qualitative references, (3) the perceived intensity of each sensory attribute, rated on an absolute (rather than relative basis) and anchored to specific references, and (4) statistical evaluation of the descriptive data, usually with analysis of variance (see Chapter 7 on Statistics) and multivariate data analysis.

Spectrum Method: Case Study

Objective

A meat processing company wanted to determine if there was a difference in appearance, flavor, and texture of a dried meat product manufactured with the current processing procedure versus a product manufactured with a new procedure that eliminated one processing step.

Method

The Spectrum Descriptive Analysis method for identifying and rating intensity was used to evaluate samples manufactured using both the current and the new method. The company wanted a standard scale, such as the universal scale used in Spectrum analysis (0 = none to 15 = very strong with reference intensities noted) in order to compare to other products from other studies.

Twelve highly trained, experienced Spectrum method respondents evaluated the seven appearance, ten flavor, and twelve texture attributes. A total of six test samples, four current and two made with the new manufacturing procedure, were evaluated for intensity of each characteristic. Samples were sliced to uniform thickness. Respondents received 25 slices of each product for evaluation: five for appearance, ten for flavor, and ten for texture. Samples were evaluated individually in random order on the 15-point Spectrum scale divided into tenths.

Results

The following data represent one attribute for each of the appearance, flavor, and texture spectrums.

	Current	Test	Current	Current	Test	Current
·Color intensity	13.5	8.0	14.3	12.0	9.0	13.5
Garlic	11.0	7.0	10.0	9.8	7.0	9.2
Cohesive	10.0	7.0	9.2	9.5	7.5	10.0

The samples manufactured using the current process had intensity ratings that were very similar for appearance, including color. The samples produced with the new manufacturing procedures were, however, very different from the current process. For flavor, the "current" samples differed in garlic, indicating some differences in process control, but were similar for all other characteristics. The "test" processes were different in many characteristics. For texture, samples from "control" and "test" processes were consistent within process and similar to each other for all characteristics except hardness, cohesive, and fibrous when the "control" product was higher than "new."

Conclusions

Based on the final Spectrum intensity ratings of the attributes, the results indicate a difference in the dried meat products produced with the different processes. The "control" product was typical of regular production. The "new" process apparently eliminated one step that was important to the final product characteristics. The current product was consistent except for "garlic" that varied slightly in the control procedure.

General Rating Scale for Attribute Intensity

This method is actually a commonly used "generic" method based on a design to measure the perceived intensity of some specified characteristic(s) or attribute(s) of a material. The dimension of evaluation may be specific or general (for example, hydrogen sulfide odor or sweetness of a beverage). It may be used with any material or product and for any attribute which can be clearly understood by the respondents.

Respondents, who have been specifically trained and instructed in regard to the attributes to be evaluated, are served a series of samples. This method is useful in evaluating a single sample or series of samples. Each sample is rated for intensity on an interval scale such as alternate points anchored as follows: none, slight, moderate, large, and extreme. When evaluating more than one attribute, a scale for each attribute is necessary. This method is commonly used in many industries, but especially in those, such as the meat industry, which often focus on only a few attributes (for example, tenderness, juiciness, meaty, warmed-over flavor).

A list of the sensory attributes that may apply to the product type is developed. Samples are examined by the respondents who indicate those characteristics which they believe apply. Sometimes the intensities of characteristics are also indicated.

The first step is the development of the list of terms. The length and scope of the list may vary with the test purpose. It may include only a limited number of attributes or characteristics, such as those which are most likely to occur or those the experimenter is interested in, or it may expand to include every characteristic that might conceivably apply.

A printed list is provided, usually with the attributes grouped according to some logical scheme, for example, by odor, texture, appearance, etc. Samples are served monadically and a large amount of sample may be required if the list is long and the respondents need to retest the sample often. The respondents go through the list and check those attributes that are present. Results are stated in terms of the percentage of times each attribute is checked. McNemar's test commonly is used to determine differences between number of times attributes are perceived in the present products, if that is important. After the list has been developed a score sheet can be designed based on the test objective. Once the score sheet has been developed the panel uses this score sheet to determine the intensity of each attribute or characteristic that is present in the test products. Analysis of variance is used to determine whether differences occur in ratings of products.

General Rating Scale Method: Case Study

Objective

To determine the degree to which two meat products differ over time in oxidative off-notes. The data will be used to determine correlations with instrumental measures. The study will be conducted on products containing either of two antioxidants or a blind control with no additive.

Method

A 15 centimeter line scale divided into 16 points (0 to 15) was chosen for this test to measure the attribute "cardboardy/oxidized." Anchor points were "none" and "extreme."

This method was chosen to give the experimenter a measure of the intensity of the specific off-note that was expected in the meat products. It was decided in advance that testing would continue beyond the point of distinguishable difference for that specific attribute in order to plot a curvilinear relationship of intensity and storage time. Therefore, the difference tests such as triangle, paired difference, and duo trio were not suitable. The line scale method also allows comparison of the three products using analysis of variance.

Respondents were recruited, screened for the ability to detect the off-note, and then trained to recognize cardboardy/oxidized and to quantify it.

Data were analyzed using analysis of variance (see Chapter 7 on Statistics).

Results

	Control	Treatment A	Treatment B	Significant Differences[a]
Week 0	1.5	2.0	1.7	NSD
Week 2	5.0	3.0	3.1	C A B
Week 4	9.7	4.2	7.6	C B A
Week 6	14.3	3.9	7.9	C B A

[a]NSD = not significantly different; treatments connected by common underscoring are not significantly different from each other but are different from products not underlined together in cardboard/oxidized rating.

Recommendation

We conclude that Treatment A is more effective than Treatment B in controlling the oxidative rancidity from a flavor standpoint. Additional research will be conducted to verify the acceptability of the product and establish a new "pull by" date prior to making the formulation change.

Time-Intensity

All sensations perceived in food beverages systems show change in intensity over time as the food is exposed to physical, thermal, chemical, and dilution effects in the mouth and nasal passages. However, most sensory procedures require the respondent to provide a single intensity response representing the entire perceptual experience prior to swallowing. This averaged response can result in the loss of valuable information related to onset and duration of attributes important to product acceptance.

In order to measure the temporal aspects of sensory perception, a technique is required that measures sensory intensity at multiple time points during the entire exposure period. The techniques that measure changes with time in the intensity of a sensation are referred to generally as time-intensity methods.

The accurate measurement of intensity changes require highly trained respondents, generally drawn from a pool of descriptive respondents familiar with the sensation being measured, and extensively trained in the data collection technique. The extension of this methodology to measure Hedonic responses over time has been explored, but classic time-intensity methodology refers to the measurement of attribute intensity.

There are three key means of collecting time-intensity data. Originally data were collected on traditional paper ballots, with some sort of visual or verbal cue used to elicit responses at selected time intervals. Another common technique is the use of a strip chart recorder to continuously collect intensity ratings as the respondent moves a pen across an intensity scale as the paper moves at a set rate. With the advent of computerized systems, responses often are collected with a variety of input devices (for example, joystick, potentiometer, mouse) and responses can be tracked and measured by the microprocessor.

The time-intensity technique is generally limited to the measurement of a single attribute during the exposure period. Infrequent or lengthy time intervals can allow for multiple attributes to be rated, although only certain data collection devices will allow for this option.

The panel protocol can vary greatly, and needs to be well defined before initiating a time-intensity study. Issues surrounding the stimulus include such items as application, length, length of exposure before expectoration/swallowing, total response time, and sample manipulation instructions. The response issues include choice of scale, discrete or continuous data collection, number of time points to collect data, and use of reference points.

Data analysis is handled generally by extracting selected parameters such as maximum intensity, time to maximum intensity, duration, and area under the curve, and applying standard statistical analyses used for descriptive data.

Transformation of the data and the development of summary curves are complicated by the individual nature of each respondent's curve and currently are under investigation by many researchers. No one technique has yet been established, and the field of time-intensity research is rapidly evolving.

Many different products can benefit from time-intensity measurements, in both food and nonfood categories. Examples include short-time responses such as onset of sweetness in a beverage, long-term responses such as elasticity changes in chewing gum, effectiveness of skin cream over time, and longevity of lather in a shampoo.

Bibliography

Methods

Brandt, M. A., Skinner, E. Z., and Coleman, J. A., "Texture Profile Methods," *Journal of Food Science,* Vol. 28, 1963, pp. 404–409.

Caul, J. F., Vol. 7, "The Profile Method of Flavor Analysis," *Advances in Food Research,* E. M. Mrak and G. F. Stewart, Eds., Academic Press, New York, 1957, pp. 1–40.

Civille, G. V. and Szcznesniak, S., "Guidelines to Training a Texture Profile Panel," *Journal of Textural Studies,* Vol. 4, 1973, pp. 204–223.

Civille, G. V. and Lawless, H. T., "The Importance of Language in Describing Perceptions," *Journal of Sensory Studies,* Vol. 1, 1986, pp. 203–215.

Cross, H. R., Moen, R., and Stanfield, M. S., "Training and Testing of Judges for Sensory Analysis of Meat Quality," *Food Technology,* Vol. 32, No. 7, 1978, pp. 48–54.

Einstein, M. A., "Descriptive Techniques and Their Hybridization," *Sensory Theory and Applications in Foods, Chapter 11,* H. T. Lawless and B. P. Kelin, Eds., Marcel Dekker, New York, 1991, pp. 317–338.

Halpern, B. P., "More Than Meets the Tongue: Temporal Characteristics or Taste Intensity and Quality," *Sensory Science Theory and Applications, Chapter 2,* H. T. Lawless and B. P. Klein, Eds., Marcel Dekker, New York, 1991, pp. 37–106.

Lee, W. E. III and Pangborn, R. M., "Time-Intensity: The Temporal Aspects of Sensory Perception," *Food Technology,* Vol. 40, No. 11, 1986, pp. 71–78, 82.

Meilgaard, C. C., "Descriptive Analysis Techniques, V. Designing a Descriptive Procedure: The Spectrum™ Method," pp. 196–199. *Chapter 8,* "Selection and Training of Panel Members," pp. 152–185, *Sensory Evaluation Techniques, Chapter 9,* CRC Press, Boca Raton, FL, 1991.

Noble, A. C., Matysiak, N. L., and Bonnans, S., "Factors Affecting the Time-Intensity Parameters of Sweetness," *Food Technology,* Vol. 45, No. 11, 1991, pp. 121–124, 126.

Sjostrom, L. B., Cairncross, S. E., and Caul, J. F., "Methodology of the Flavor Profile," *Food Technology,* Vol. 11, No. 9, Sept. 1957, pp. 20–25.

Stone, H., Sidel, J. L., Oliver, S., Woolsey, A., and Singleton, R. C., "Sensory Evaluation by Quantitative Descriptive Analysis," *Food Technology,* Vol. 28, No. 11, Nov. 1974, pp. 25–34.

Stone, H., Sidel, J. L., and Bloomquist, J., "Quantitative Descriptive Analysis," *Cereal Foods World,* Vol. 25, No. 10, 1980, pp. 642–644.

Applications

Abbott, J. A., Watada, A. E., and Massie, D. R., "Sensory and Instrument Measurement of Apple Texture," *Journal of American Society for Horticultural Science,* Vol. 109, No. 2, 1984, pp. 221–228.

Bramesco, N. P. and Setser, C. S., "Application of Sensory Texture Profiling to Baked Products: Some Considerations for Evaluation, Definition of Parameters, and Reference Products," *Journal of Textural Studies,* Vol. 21, 1990, pp. 235–251.

Caul, J. F. and Vaden, A. G., "Flavor of White Bread as It Ages," *Bakers Digest,* Vol. 46, No. 1, 1972, pp. 39, 42–43, 60.

Chambers, E. IV, Bowers, J. R., and Smith, E. A., "Flavor of Cooked, Ground Turkey Patties with Added Sodium Tripolphosphate as Perceived by Sensory Panels with Differing Phosphate Sensitivity," *Journal of Food Science,* Vol. 57, No. 2, 1992, pp. 521–523.

Chambers, E. IV and Robel, A., "Sensory Characteristics of Selected Species of Freshwater Fish in Retail Distribution," *Journal of Food Science,* Vol. 58, No. 3, 1993, pp. 508–512, 561.

Chang, C. and Chambers, E. IV, "Flavor Characterization of Breads Made From Hard Red Winter Wheat and Hard White Winter Wheat," *Cereal Chamistry,* Vol. 69, No. 5, 1992, pp. 556–559.

Civille, G. V. and Dus, C. A., "Development of Terminology to Describe the Handfeel Properties of Paper and Fabrics," *Journal of Sensory Studies,* Vol. 5, 1990, pp. 19–32.

Civille, G. V. and Liska, I. H., "Modifactions and Applications to Foods of the General Foods Sensory Texture Profile Technique," *Journal of Textural Studies,* Vol. 6, 1975, pp. 19–31.

Clapperton, J. F., "Derviation of a Profile Method for Sensory Analysis of Beer Flavor," *Journal of the Institute of Brewing,* Vol. 79, 1973, pp. 495–508.

Clapperton, J. F., "Sensory Characterisation of the Flavour of Beer," *Progress in Flavor Research, 2nd edition, Chapter 1,* D. G. Land, Ed., Applied Science, London, 1979, pp. 1–14.

Gardze, C., Bowers, J. A., and Caul, J. F., "Effect of Salt and Textured Soy Level on Sensory Characteristics of Beef Patties," *Journal of Food Science,* Vol. 44, 1979, pp. 460–464.

Gillette, M., "Applications of Descriptive Analysis," *Journal of Food Protection,* Vol. 47, No. 5, 1984, pp. 403–409.

Gupta, S. K., Karahadian, C., and Lindsay, R. C., "Effect of Emulsifier Salts on Textural and Flavor Properties of Processed Cheeses," *Journal of Dairy Science,* Vol. 67, 1984, pp. 764–778.

Heisserer, D. M. and Chambers, E. IV, "Determination of the Sensory Flavor Attributes of Aged Natural Cheese," *Journal of Sensory Studies,* Vol. 8, 1993, pp. 121–132.

Johnsen, P. B. and Civille, G. V., "A Standardization Lexicon of Meat WOF Descriptors," *Journal of Sensory Studies,* Vol. 1, 1986, pp. 99–104.

Johnsen, P. B., Civille, G. V., and Vercellotti, J. R., "A Lexicon of Pond-Raised Catfish Flavor Descriptors," *Journal of Sensory Studies,* Vol. 2, 1987, pp. 85–91.

Johnsen, P. B., Civille, G. V., Vercellotti, J. R., Sanders, T. H., and Dus, C. A., "Development of a Lexicon for the Description of Peanut Flavor," *Journal of Sensory Studies*, Vol. 3, 1988, pp. 9–17.

Lyon, B. G., "Development of Chicken Flavor Descriptive Attribute Terms Aided by Multivariate Statistical Procedures," *Journal of Sensory Studies*, Vol. 2, 1987, pp. 55–67.

Kokini, J. L., Poole, M., Mason, P., Miller, S., and Stier, E. F., "Identification of Key Textural Attributes of Fluid and Semi-Solid Foods Using Regression Analysis," *Journal of Food Science*, Vol. 49, 1984, pp. 47–51.

Maligalig, L. L., Caul, J. F., and Tiemeier, O. W., "Aroma and Flavor of Farm-Raised Channel Catfish: Effects of Pond Condition, Storage, and Diet," *Food Product and Development*, Vol. 7, No. 5, 1973, p. 4.

Mecredy, J. M., Sonnemann, J. C., and Lehmann, S. J., "Sensory Profiling of Beer by a Modified QDA Method," *Food Technology*, Vol. 28, No. 11, 1974, pp. 36–41.

Moore, L. J. and Shoemaker, C. F., "Sensory Textural Properties of Stabilized Ice Cream," *Journal of Food Science*, Vol. 46, No. 2, 1981, pp. 399–402, 499.

Muñoz, A. M., Pangborn, R. M., and Noble, A. C., "Sensory and Mechanical Attributes of Gel Texture. I. Effect of Gelatin Concentration," *Journal of Texture Studies*, Vol 17, 1986, pp. 1–16.

Muñoz, A. M., Pangborn, R. M., and Noble, A. C., "Sensory and Mechanical Attributes of Gel Texture. II. Gelatin, Sodium Alginate and Kappa-Carrageenan Gels," *Journal of Texture Studies*, Vol. 17, 1986, pp. 17–36.

Noble, A. C., "Precision and Communication: Descriptive Analysis of Wine," *1984 Wine Industry Technical Symposium*, 1984, pp. 33–41.

Ott, D. B., Edwards, C. L., and Palmer, S. J., "Perceived Taste Intensity and Duration of Nutritive and Nonnutritive Sweeteners in Water Using Time-Intensity (T-I) Evaluations," *Journal of Food Science*, Vol. 56, 1991, p. 535.

Powers, N. L. and Pangborn, R. M., "Descriptive Analysis of the Sensory Properties of Beverages and Gelatins Containing Sucrose or Synthetic Sweeteners," *Journal of Food Science*, Vol. 43, pp. 47–51.

Resurrection, A. V. A. and Shewfelt, R. L., "Relationships Between Sensory Attributes and Objective Measurements of Postharvest Quality of Tomatoes," *Journal of Food Science*, Vol. 50, 1985, pp. 1242–1245.

Smith, E. A., Chambers, E. IV, and Colley, S., "Development of Vocabulary and References for Describing Off-Odors in Raw Drains," *Cereal Foods World*, Vol. 39, No. 7, July 1994, pp. 496–499.

Szczesniak, A. S., "Classification of Textural Characteristics," *Journal of Food Science*, Vol. 28, 1963, pp. 385–389.

Szczesniak, A. S., Brandt, M. A., and Friedman, H. H., "Development of Standard Rating Scales for Mechanical Parameters of Texture and Correlation Between the Objective and the Sensory Methods of Texture Evaluation," *Journal of Food Science*, Vol. 28, 1963, pp. 397–403.

Chapter 6—Affective Testing

Affective testing is used to determine preference, liking, or attitudes about products and other materials. Its use in research situations often is limited to providing guidance and direction to developers and researchers. The scope of this manual does not include large scale marketing research tests used for making final decisions about product sales, marketing, and positioning although many of the same techniques are used.

Affective research guidance testing is conducted almost exclusively with naive respondents (consumers). Although "bench top" screening occurs with researchers and employees and should follow the same guidelines as for consumers, consumer input is necessary and should be obtained for most tests.

Most affective testing that is conducted by sensory groups usually is quantitative in nature, that is, the tests measure how much or how many. Qualitative testing, such as focus groups and in-depth interviews, is conducted both by sensory groups and marketing research but is beyond the scope of this manual. Typical quantitative tests include the hedonic scale method that measures degree of liking, or preference testing that measures how many people prefer one product to another.

Hedonic Scale Method

This is a rating scale method of measuring the level of liking for products where affective tone is important. The method relies on the naive or untrained respondent's capacity to report, directly and reliably, their feelings of like or dislike within the context of the test. An important aspect of the method is that it is used with untrained people, although a minimum level of verbal ability is required for adequate performance.

Samples are presented monadically, sequentially, or in groups, and the respondent is told to decide how much he likes or dislikes each sample and to mark the scales accordingly. The essence of the method is its simplicity. Instructions to the respondents are restricted to procedures. No attempt is made to direct the actual response. The respondent is allowed to make inferences about the meaning of the scale categories and self-determine how the scale will be used to express the respondents feelings about the samples. A separate printed scale usually is provided for each sample presented in the test session.

Many different forms of Hedonic scales may be used without major effect on the value of the results as long as the essential feature of the verbal anchoring of successive categories is retained. The most common hedonic scales are the nine- and seven-point category scales. Variation in the number of categories is acceptable with the use of fewer than five categories not recommended. Alternate forms of scales are the line-scale and the replacement of the verbal category scale with caricatures representing degrees of pleasure and displeasure (often referred to as the Smiley scale). Although the relative measures tend to remain

73

constant, variations in scale form are likely to cause changes in the distributions of responses and, consequently, in such statistical parameters as means and variances.

The levels of rating obtained on the Hedonic scale may be affected by many factors other than the quality of the test samples, such as, characteristics of the respondents or the test situation, and transitory attitudes or expectations of the respondents. Consequently, one should be extremely cautious about making inferences on the basis of comparisons obtained in separate experiments. This is permissible only when large numbers of respondents have participated and test conditions have been consistently maintained. The relative differences in liking among samples tested together tend to be consistent across a series of test replications.

A common decision that must be made is whether or not to provide one product per consumer or whether to provide a series of products (two or more) to each consumer. Monodic or multiple test designs are solely based on the objective of the test. Although there is no one correct answer, it may be easier to find differences in liking if multiple samples are evaluated by each consumer. Also, it is almost always more efficient to provide consumers more than one sample and few problems are encountered if that is done. However, the following considerations must be made:

1. First order bias sometimes exists and consumers may consistently score the first product higher or lower than other products regardless of what product is evaluated. Therefore, order of sample presentation is critical.

2. It may be helpful to carry out an analysis on only the data of first samples to determine if major findings would change. However, caution needs to be exercised in doing this because the statistical test will be less sensitive because fewer total number of evaluations are included in the test making the statistical test less sensitive.

3. In some situations a first sample that serves as a "warm up" may be used in the test, but not included in the analysis.

Hedonic Scale Method: Case Study

Objective

Determine if adding vanillin improves acceptability of a beverage product.

Test Method

The Hedonic scale was selected for this study because it will show whether adding vanillin increases acceptance with consumers. One hundred consumers were selected who consume beverages in the category to be tested. Each consumer tested both samples in a sequential monadic test (a sample was presented, scored and removed before the second sample was given). The order of presentation was balanced so that half of the consumers received the "control" first and half received the "vanillin" treatment first. Results were analyzed by analysis of variance or paired t-test (see Chapter 7 on Statistics).

Results

Hedonic Attribute	Total (n = 100)		
	Vanillin		Control
Overall liking	6.7	*	5.7
Liking of appearance	6.5	*	5.9
Liking of color	6.6	*	5.9
Liking of flavor	6.6	**	5.5
Liking of sweetness	6.7	NS	6.5
Liking of texture	6.8	NS	6.4

NS = not significant
* = $P \leq 0.05$ indicates a significant difference at 95% confidence level.
** = $P \leq 0.01$ indicates a significant difference at 99% confidence level.
The analysis indicated that the product with added vanillin is liked significantly more than control overall and for appearance, color, and flavor. Therefore, adding vanillin does improve the product.

Recommendation

Based on these sensory data, it is recommended that adding vanillin be considered further as an improvement for this product.

Paired Preference Test

One of the most common methods of affective testing is the paired-preference test. The test is used extensively for determining which of two samples is better. It is a forced-choice method and consumers are not allowed to give a "no preference" response.

The test is simple in principle. Two samples are presented to a naive respondent who is asked to choose the one that he or she prefers. The samples usually are presented simultaneously and respondents directly compare the samples, although sequential presentation is sometimes done if the samples have a characteristic that would prevent multiple sampling in a single session.

Order of presentation must be balanced in preference testing because position biases often are noted. That "rule" must not be violated, except in extremely unusual circumstances, because the position bias often is so strong that results likely will be incorrect if presentation is not balanced.

Because preference testing usually asks the respondent to evaluate the product on a total basis, this type of testing can be especially susceptible to unintentional biases. Problems such as different serving temperatures, different amounts in the testing container; slight differences in manufacturing tolerances for color, fragrance, size, or other variables; and unintended biases caused by seemingly slight differences in presentation such as sitting one sample slightly closer to the respondent all may cause the overall appeal of a sample to change. As with all testing, care must be exercised to control the test procedures.

Paired Preference Test: Case Study

Objective

Determine whether a company's graham cracker or its major competitor is preferred by consumers.

Test Method

Paired preference was used to determine which graham cracker was the preferred graham cracker because a single test of preference was all the information that was needed. Four hundred consumers were randomly selected for the test. The samples were presented simultaneously coded with 3-digit random codes and consumers were instructed to test the sample on the left first and then the sample on the right. The serving order was balanced with half the consumers sampling the company's product first and the other half sampling the competitive product first. Results were analyzed by computing a z-score (that is, the normal approximation to the binomial distribution).

Results

Product	# Preferring	Percent	z
Company	249	62.3	4.9
Competitor	151	37.8	

The z-score was computed as

$$z = \frac{x - n(p_0)}{\sqrt{n(p_0)(1 - p_0)}}$$

where $p_0 = 1/2$, the null hypothesis value corresponding to no preference. The test statistic z follows a standard normal distribution.

$$= \frac{249 - 400(1/2)}{\sqrt{400(1/2)(1(1/2))}} = 49/10 = 4.9$$

The critical value of the standard normal are the same as those of the Student's t distribution with α degrees of freedom. Entering the last row of the Student's table, Chapter 7, Table 4, one finds that $z = 4.9$ exceeds the $\alpha = 0.01$ critical value of $t_\alpha = 2.326$.

Recommendations

The company's product is the preferred graham cracker.

Bibliography

Methods

Bengston, R. and Brenner, H., "Product Test Results Using Three Different Methodologies," *Journal of Marketing Research*, Vol. 37, No. 1, 1965, pp. 49–53.

Birch, L. L., "Dimensions of Preschool Children's Food Preferences: One Result of This Study Points to the Feasibility of Obtaining Preference Data Directly from Young Children," *Journal of Nutrition Education*, Vol. 11, No. 2, April–June 1979, pp. 77–80.

Coleman, J. A., "Measuring Consumer Acceptance of Foods and Beverages," *Food Technology*, Vol. 18, No. 11, 1964, pp. 53–54.

Daillant, B. and Issanchou, S., "Most Preferred Level of Sugar: Rapid Measure and Consumption Methods for Measuring Consumer Preference," *Journal of Sensory Studies*, Vol. 6, No. 3, 1991, pp. 131–144.

Kamen, J. M., Peryam, D. R., Peryam, D. B., and Kroll, B. J., "Hedonic Differences as a Function of Number of Samples Evaluated," *Journal of Food Science*, Vol. 34, 1969, pp. 475–479.

Moskowitz, H. R., Jacobs, B. E., and Neil, L., "Product Response Segmentation and the Analysis of Individual Differences in Liking," *Journal of Food Quality*, Vol. 8, No. 2/3, 1985, pp. 169–181.

Peryam, D. R. and Pilgrim, F. J., "Hedonic Scale Method of Measuring Food Preferences," *Food Technology*, Vol. 11, No. 9, 1957, pp. 9–14.

Peryam, D. R. and Gutman, N. J., "Variation in Preference Ratings for Foods Served at Meals," *Food Technology*, Vol. 12, No. 1, 1958, pp. 30–33.

Pilgrim, F. J. and Kenneth, W., "Comparative Sensitivity of Rating Scale and Paired Comparison Methods for Measuring Consumer Preference," *Food Technology*, Vol. 9, 1955, pp. 385–387.

Roessler, E. B., Pangborn, R. M., Sidel, J. L., and Stone, H., "Expanded Statistical Tables for Estimating Significance in Paired-Preference, Paired-Difference, Duo-Trio and Triangle Tests," *Journal of Food Science*, Vol. 43, 1978, pp. 940–947.

Simone, M. and Pangborn, R. M., "Consumer Acceptance Methodology: One vs. Two Samples," *Food Technology*, Vol. 11, No. 9, 1957, pp. 25–29.

Schutz, H. G., "A Food Action Rating Scale for Measuring Food Acceptance," *Journal of Food Science*, Vol. 30, 1965, pp. 365–374.

Spaeth, E. E., Chambers, E. IV, and Schwenke, J. R., "A Comparison of Acceptability Scaling Methods for Use with Children," *Product Testing with Special Consumer Populations for Research Guidance*, L. S. Wu, and A. D. Gelinas, Eds., American Society for Testing and Materials, Philadelphia, 1992, pp. 65–77.

Applications

Chambers, L., Chambers, E. IV, and Bowers, J. R., "Consumer Acceptability of Cooked Stored Ground Turkey Patties with Differing Levels of Phosphate," *Journal of Food Science*, Vol. 57, No. 4, 1992, pp. 1026–1028.

Moskowitz, H. R., Wolfe, K., and Beck, C., "Sweetness and Acceptance Optimization in Cola Flavored Beverages Using Combinations of Artificial Sweeteners—a Psychophysical Approach," *Journal of Food Quality*, Vol. 2, 1978, pp. 17–26.

Pangborn, R. M. and Nickerson, T. A., "The Influence of Sugar in Ice Cream. II. Consumer Preferences for Strawberry Ice Cream," *Food Technology*, Vol. 13, No. 2, 1959, pp. 107–109.

Pangborn, R. M., Sherman, L., Simone, M., and Luh, B. S., "Freestone Peaches. I. Effect of Sucrose, Citric Acid, and Corn Syrup on Consumer Acceptance," *Food Technology*, Vol. 13, No. 8, 1959, pp. 444–447.

Griffin, R. and Stauffer, L., "Product Optimization in Central-Location Testing and Subsequent Validation and Calibration in Home-Use Testing," *Journal of Sensory Studies*, Vol. 5, 1990, pp. 231–240.

Randall, C. J. and Larmond, E., "Effect of Method of Comminution (Flake-Cutting and Grinding) on the Acceptability and Quality of Hamburger Patties," *Journal of Food Science*, Vol. 42, No. 3, 1977, pp. 728–730.

White, F. D., Resurreccion, A. V. A., and Lillard, D. A., "Effect of Warmed Over Flavor on Consumer Acceptance and Purchase of Precooked Top Round Steaks," *Journal of Food Science*, Vol. 53, No. 5, 1988, pp. 1251–1257.

Chapter 7—Statistical Procedures

This section is included for the convenience of the readers and users of this manual. The primary objective of this section is to provide the researcher who has a limited knowledge of statistics with tools to design studies and to analyze and interpret the results from those studies. It presents the statistical methods needed to analyze the data obtained and to determine the statistical significance of differences found when using the methods described in this manual. Statistical significance will occur when the observed differences among products or panels are greater than the observed differences within products or panels. It is important to note that a statistically significant difference does not necessarily imply an important difference or a difference with practical significance. Similarly, the absence of a statistically significant difference does not mean that one does not exist, particularly if small sample sizes are used. This section also includes a glossary of some frequently encountered statistical terms and symbols. Several references are provided for those who have more complicated problems, who wish to obtain more detail, or who wish to become more generally proficient in statistics.

A. Glossary of Statistical Terms and Symbols

This glossary contains a number of definitions for frequently encountered statistical terms and symbols. It is not meant to be all inclusive. In the bibliography of this manual are several statistical texts which should be consulted for more extensive definitions and explanations. Formulas and symbols are included in the definitions where they are appropriate. An illustration of some common operations on two arbitrary data sets is included to aid in using this section.

1. Definitions

Alternate Hypothesis—See section on "Hypothesis Testing."
Symbol H_1

Confidence Interval—This is the interval within which a population value is expected to be found with some specified probability. The usual statement is "the 95% confidence interval for x is $x \pm k$." The statement is interpreted as saying that there is a 95% probability that the value of x will be between $(x - k)$ and $(x + k)$. Note that there is a relationship to "statistical significance" since the statement infers that less than 5% of the time the value of x will be outside of the confidence interval.

Degrees of Freedom—This is a difficult concept related to the independence of observations. A complete discussion is beyond the scope of this manual. However, the basic meaning can be shown by the following. If the mean of n observations is known, then specifying the values of any $n - 1$ of the observations fixes the

79

value of the remaining observation and the set is said to have $n - 1$ degrees of freedom. For example, if the mean of 6 observations is 3.5 and we know that 5 of the observations are 2, 5, 3, 6, 3 then the remaining observation must be (6 · 3.5) − 2 − 5 − 3 − 6 − 3 = 2. The degrees of freedom are 5 or $n - 1$. Also see the example data sets and the section on "hypothesis testing."

Geometric Mean—The geometric mean of a set of n-numbers is the Nth root of the cumulative product of the numbers. Another way of defining the geometric mean is the antilog of the arithmetic mean of the logarithms of the numbers in the set. This is usually easier to calculate. Note that a geometric mean may be calculated only for data sets where all values are positive.

Symbol $\bar{x}_g$

Formula $\bar{x}_g = (x_1 \cdot x_2 \cdot x_3 \cdot \ldots x_n)^{1/n}$

Calculation formula

$$\bar{x}_g = \text{Antilog} \frac{(\log(x_1) + \log(x_2) + \log(x_3) + \cdots \log(x_n))}{n}$$

Interval Data—Numbers used to denote a distance or location on a known continuous scale with a zero point that is usually arbitrary.

Examples: time or temperature

Mean—The arithmetic average of a set of observed values.

Symbol $\bar{x}$ (μ is used for the population mean)

Formula $\bar{x} = \dfrac{\Sigma x}{n}$

where

Σx = sum of the individual values and
n = the number of individual values.

Median—The midpoint of a set of observed values which have been ordered from the lowest to the highest. Exactly half the values are higher than the median and half are lower. See example data sets.

Nominal Data—Numbers or symbols used to denote membership in a group or class.

Examples: Zip codes, male/female, area codes

Null Hypothesis—See section on "Hypothesis Testing"

Symbol H_o

Probability Distribution—A mathematical equation that relates the value of an observation (for example, an individual's height) to the likelihood of observing that value.

One-Sided and Two-Sided Hypothesis Test—See section on "Hypothesis Testing."

Ordinal Data—Numbers used to denote a ranking within or between groups or classes.
  Examples: preference, socioeconomic status

p-Value—The probability associated with some observation or statistic.

Ratio Data—A special case of interval data where a true zero exists.
  Examples: mass, volume, density

Random Sample—A sample taken from a population in such a way as to give each individual in the population an equal chance of being selected.

Sample—A subset of observed values from a population of values.

Standard Deviation—The square root of the variance.
  Symbol SEM ($s_{\bar{x}}$ is sometimes used)
  Formula SEM $= \dfrac{s}{\sqrt{n}}$

Statistic—A function of the observed values in a sample. Statistics are used to estimate the population values (for example, x estimates the population mean, μ). Statistics are also used to test hypotheses (for example, x or the t-test).

Statistical Significance—See section on "Hypothesis Testing."

Subscripts—Subscripts are used to identify members of a set of data. For example: $x_1, x_2, x_3 \ldots x_n$. They may also be used to identify different sets of data such as X_A and X_B

Variance—A measure of the scatter or dispersion of a set of observed values about the mean of the set.
  Symbol s^2 (σ^2 is used for the population variance)
  Formula $s^2 = \dfrac{\Sigma(x - \bar{x})^2}{n - 1}$

  Calculation formula $s^2 = \dfrac{\Sigma x^2 - \dfrac{(\Sigma x)^2}{n}}{(n - 1)}$

2. Some Other Common Symbols

  d The difference between two values.
  $\bar{d}$ The mean difference between two sets of paired values.
  p, q The two values of proportion such that $q = 1 - p$.
  α The Type I error probability (see "Statistical Errors" section).
  β The Type II error probability (see "Statistical Errors" section).

	Set A	Set A^2	Set B	Set B^2	A − B	(A − B)^2
		Illustrative Examples of Some Statistical Calculations				
X_1	5	25	3	9	2	4
X_2	6	36	1	1	5	25
X_3	4	16	4	16	0	0
X_4	3	9	5	25	−2	4
X_5	5	25	6	36	−1	1
X_6	6	36	4	16	2	4
X_7	4	16	2	4	2	4
X_8	4	16	5	25	−1	1
X_9	3	9	4	16	−1	1
X_{10}	7	49	3	9	4	16
Sum	47	237	37	157	10	60
n	10		10		10	
Median	4.5		4		1	

Mean (sum/n)	4.7	3.7	1.0
Variance	$237 - \dfrac{(47 * 47)}{10}$	$157 - \dfrac{(37 * 37)}{10}$	$60 - \dfrac{(10 * 10)}{10}$
	$\overline{\qquad(10 - 1)\qquad}$	$\overline{\qquad(10 - 1)\qquad}$	$\overline{\qquad(10 - 1)\qquad}$
	1.789	2.233	5.556
Standard deviation	$\sqrt{1.789}$	$\sqrt{2.233}$	$\sqrt{5.556}$
	1.337	1.494	2.357
SEM	$\dfrac{1.337}{\sqrt{10}}$	$\dfrac{1.494}{\sqrt{10}}$	$\dfrac{2.357}{\sqrt{10}}$
	0.423	0.472	0.745

B. Hypothesis Testing

Hypothesis testing is an approach for drawing conclusions about a population, as a whole, based on the information contained in a sample of items from that population. Hypothesis testing is used, for example, to determine if some parameter of interest has a particular value (for example, that the probability of a correct response in a duo-trio test is 50%) or to compare two or more items based on some measurement of interest (for example, that sample A has the same sweetness intensity as sample B).

The Null and Alternative Hypotheses

The first step in hypothesis testing is to develop the null hypothesis and the alternative hypothesis. The null hypothesis states the conditions that are assumed to exist before the study is run. It serves as the baseline in the calculation of test statistics and their associated probabilities (that is, p-values). For a duo-trio test the null hypothesis is H_0: $P_c = 0.50$ (where P_c is the probability of correctly selecting the odd sample)—that is, in the absence of any perceptible difference between two samples, there is only a 50:50 chance of picking the matching samples. For comparing two samples, A and B, based on some measurement, the null hypothesis is H_0: $\mu_A = \mu_B$. That is, there is no difference between the samples, on the average. The alternative hypothesis states the conditions that are of interest to the investigator if the null hypothesis is not true. For a duo-trio test the alternative hypothesis is H_1: $P_c > 0.50$. That is, if there is a perceptible difference between the two samples, the chance of picking the odd sample is greater than 50%. For comparing two samples, A and B, based on some measurement, one of three alternative hypotheses will be appropriate: H_1: $\mu_A < \mu_B$, H_1: $\mu_A > \mu_B$, H_1: $\mu_A \neq \mu_B$.

One-Sided and Two-Sided Alternative Hypotheses

Where the null hypothesis is generally arrived at by default, serious attention must be paid to developing the alternative hypothesis to ensure that it accurately summarizes the prior interest of the investigator. When comparing two samples, for example, if the investigator is not interested in the direction of the difference, but only that one exists, then the alternative hypothesis is two-sided (for example, H_1: $\mu_A \neq \mu_B$). If, on the other hand, the investigator is specifically interested in the direction of the difference and the appropriate test has been conducted based on that interest, then the alternative hypothesis is one-sided (for example, H_1: $\mu_A < \mu_B$ or H_1: $\mu_A > \mu_B$). If there is uncertainty about whether the alternative hypothesis is one-sided or two-sided, guidance should be sought from some knowledgable source. If such help is not available the most conservative course is to use a two-sided alternative hypothesis.

Statistical Errors and Their Associated Probabilities

Rejecting the null hypothesis when it is true is a Type I error. The probability of making a Type I error is α. When the null hypothesis is true the probability of making the correct decision is $1 - \alpha$. Typical values for α are 0.10, 0.05, and 0.01. Failing to reject the null hypothesis when it is false (for example, failing to detect a difference that exists) is a Type II error. The probability of making a Type II error is β. The "power" of a hypothesis test is the probability of detecting a difference of a specified size; Power = $100 (1 - \beta)\%$. Typical values for β are 0.20 or less. Often only the value of α is considered when designing sensory studies (β is left to float). Sample sizes can be selected to control the size of both errors simultaneously. However, these sample sizes will be necessarily larger (sometimes prohibitively larger) than those that only control α.

In certain common sensory testing situations, called similarity tests, it is more important to control β (allowing α to float, if necessary). In a similarity test the investigator wants to minimize the chance of failing to detect a difference between samples, if one exists. An example of a similarity test is an ingredient replacement/ substitution study in which no perceptible change in the product is intended. In such cases, the value of β should be reduced to the levels commonly chosen for α (for example, 0.10, 0.05, or 0.01).

Statistical Significance

A hypothesis test yields the probability that the observed results could have occurred by chance alone. That is, the probability is computed assuming that the null hypothesis is true. If the probability is large, the null hypothesis is not rejected, because there is a reasonably large likelihood that any observed difference from what was assumed in H_0 was simply a chance occurrence (attributable solely to the fact that the results in a sample will deviate slightly from those in the total population). If, on the other hand, the probability is small (for example, less than 0.05), the null hypothesis is rejected in favor of the alternative hypothesis, because there is an unreasonably small likelihood that a difference as large as the one observed could have occurred by chance alone (in the absence of a real difference).

Two approaches are used to determine statistical significance. Either can be used because they will never yield conflicting conclusions. In the first approach, the value of the test statistic is compared to the critical value of that test statistic, using an appropriate table of critical values based on x and the sample size, n (for example, Tables 1 and 2). When the value of the test statistic is larger than the critical value in the table, the null hypothesis is rejected (at the given level of significance). The second approach uses p-values that are now commonly included in the output of statistical computer packages. The p-value is the probability of the observed results of a study occurring when the null hypothesis is true. When the p-value is smaller than the selected value of α, then the null hypothesis is rejected. P-values are slightly more informative than the test statistics because they provide a direct measure of just how unlikely the observed results are.

Example—Duo-Trio Test for the Difference Between Two Samples

Forty respondents evaluate a labeled reference sample followed by two blindly coded test samples. One of the test samples is the same as the reference. The other is different, possibly perceptibly so. The respondents are asked to select the test sample that they believe is identical to the labeled reference. The purpose of the test is to determine if people perceive a difference between the two test samples. Twenty-eight respondents correctly selected the test sample that matched the reference.

TABLE 1—*Minimum number of choices (c) required for significance for number of judgments (n) at various risk levels in a paired-comparison test where either sample may be chosen. Chance probability is 50% and the hypothesis is two-tailed.*

	(c) Risk					(c) Risk			
n	10%	5%	1%	0.1%	n	10%	5%	1%	0.1%
5	5				41	27	28	30	32
6	6	6			42	27	28	30	32
7	7	7			43	28	29	31	33
8	7	8	8		44	28	29	31	34
9	8	8	9		45	29	30	32	34
10	9	9	10		46	30	31	33	35
11	9	10	11	11	47	30	31	33	36
12	10	10	11	12	48	31	32	34	36
13	10	11	12	13	49	31	32	34	37
14	11	12	13	14	50	32	33	35	37
15	12	12	13	14					
16	12	13	14	15	52	33	34	36	39
17	13	13	15	16	54	34	35	37	40
18	13	14	15	17	56	35	36	39	41
19	14	15	16	17	58	36	37	40	42
20	15	15	17	18	60	37	39	41	44
21	15	16	17	19	62	39	40	42	45
22	16	17	18	19	64	40	41	43	46
23	16	17	19	20	66	41	42	44	47
24	17	18	19	21	68	42	43	46	48
25	18	18	20	21	70	43	44	47	50
26	18	19	20	22	72	44	45	48	51
27	19	20	21	23	74	45	46	49	52
28	19	20	22	23	76	46	48	50	53
29	20	21	22	24	78	47	49	51	54
30	20	21	23	25	80	48	50	52	56
31	21	22	24	25	82	50	51	54	57
32	22	23	24	26	84	51	52	55	58
33	22	23	25	27	86	52	53	56	59
34	23	24	25	27	88	53	54	57	60
35	23	24	26	28	90	54	55	58	61
36	24	25	27	29	92	55	56	59	63
37	24	25	27	29	94	56	57	60	64
38	25	26	28	30	96	57	59	62	65
39	26	27	28	31	98	58	60	63	66
40	26	27	29	31	100	59	61	64	67

Under the assumption of no perceptible difference between the two samples any correct selections of the test sample that matches the reference could only result from a correct guess. The chance of randomly selecting the correct test sample in a duo-trio test is 50%. Therefore, the null hypothesis for the test is H_0: $P_c = 0.50$. If there is a perceptible difference between the two test samples, then the chance of correctly selecting the one that matches the reference will increase, so the alternative hypothesis is H_1: $P_c > 0.50$. If there is no perceptible difference between the samples (that is, H_0: $P_c = 0.50$ is true), then the probability

TABLE 2—*Minimum number of correct identifications* (c) *required for significance for number of judgments* (n) *at various risk levels in two sample tests. Chance probability is 50% and the hypothesis is one-tailed.*

n	(c) Risk 10%	5%	1%	0.1%	n	(c) Risk 10%	5%	1%	0.1%
4	4				40	25	26	28	31
5	5	5			41	26	27	29	31
6	6	6			42	26	27	29	32
7	6	7	7		43	27	28	30	32
8	7	7	8		44	27	28	31	33
9	7	8	9		45	28	29	31	34
10	8	9	10	10	46	28	30	32	34
11	9	9	10	11	47	29	30	32	35
12	9	10	11	12	48	29	31	33	36
13	10	10	12	13	49	30	31	34	36
14	10	11	12	13	50	31	32	34	37
15	11	12	13	14	52	32	33	35	38
16	12	12	14	15	54	33	34	36	39
17	12	13	14	16	56	34	35	38	40
18	13	13	15	16	58	35	36	39	42
19	13	14	15	17	60	36	37	40	43
20	14	15	16	18	62	37	38	41	44
21	14	15	17	18	64	38	40	42	45
22	15	16	17	19	66	39	41	43	46
23	16	16	18	20	68	40	42	45	48
24	16	17	19	20	70	41	43	46	49
25	17	18	19	21	72	42	44	47	50
26	17	18	20	22	74	44	45	48	51
27	18	19	20	22	76	45	46	49	52
28	18	19	21	23	78	46	47	50	54
29	19	20	22	24	80	47	48	51	55
30	20	20	22	24	82	48	49	52	56
31	20	21	23	25	84	49	51	54	57
32	21	22	24	26	86	50	52	55	58
33	21	22	24	26	88	51	53	56	59
34	22	23	25	27	90	52	54	57	61
35	22	23	25	27	92	53	55	58	62
36	23	24	26	28	94	54	56	59	63
37	23	24	27	29	96	55	57	60	64
38	24	25	27	29	98	56	58	61	65
39	25	26	28	30	100	57	59	63	66

of observing 28 correct selections out of 40 in a duo-trio test is p-value $= 0.0083$. If $\alpha = 0.05$ is selected as the significance level of the test, the observed p-value is smaller than α and the null hypothesis would be rejected in favor of the alternative. It would be concluded that there is a perceptible difference between the samples. Equivalently, one could look up the critical number of correct selections in a duo-trio test of 40 respondents with $\alpha = 0.05$ in Table 2 and observe that the observed value of 28 exceeds the tabled value of 26, leading to the same conclusion.

C. Limitations and Qualifications

1. What Is Significant?

Long usage has given the 5% level ($p < 0.05$) a special status. It is the most often used level for the cutoff point between a "real" difference and one which can be accepted only with reservation, but this is convention only. Other levels can and should be used depending on the type of test and the level of risk making an incorrect recommendation. Obviously, a result which just misses the 5% level (say $P = 0.06$) is very little different from 5% and generally should not provide a completely different recommendation based on the data. The significance level used in a test is the prerogative of the experimenter and should depend upon the circumstances of the experiment and the way the results are to be used.

2. Multiple Tests of Significance

Sometimes there is a need for many tests of significance on the same data, or on related sets of observations. This is permissible; however, one must keep in mind the meaning of statistical significance. The 5% risk level implies 95 chances in 100 that the difference is "real," but also implies that there are five chances in 100 that there is no difference. As one continues to make and test hypotheses, the probability of finding one result that is "significant" just by chance, increases. For example, if just one of 20 tests attains the 5% level, there is no reason to conclude that there is anything special about the case.

3. Reliability of Results

One way of interpreting significance is in terms of what one would expect to happen if the experiment were repeated. For example, a 5% level of difference between the averages of two experimental treatments suggests that the finding of "no difference" would be unlikely; it should happen no more often than once in twenty repetitions. However, finding a significant difference does not mean that one should expect to find a difference as large or at the same level of significance whenever the experiment is replicated. It means only that one should expect to find a difference greater than zero and in the same direction as before.

4. Theoretical Basis for Statistical Analyses

Most statistical analyses are based on certain assumptions about the data. For example, most assume that the data, or random errors in the data, are normally distributed. Theoretical statisticians are often concerned about whether these assumptions are actually met, but the users of statistical computations in this manual usually need not be concerned with this.

D. Reference To Prepared Tables

The tables explained in this section give critical values for the paired comparison, duo-trio, and triangle tests at alpha risk levels of 0.10, 0.05, 0.01, and 0.001.

A 10% risk level is often adequate with noncontinuous data and where naive, nontrained respondents (consumers) instead of trained respondents are used.

1. Table 1—Significance of Paired-Comparison (Binomial) Results in Two-Tailed

(*a*) This table is for use in situations where either of the two samples may be chosen and where the chance probability is 50%. The preference test is the typical situation. It also applies to tests where comparisons have been made on the basis of other factors such as sweetness, strength, softness, etc. For two samples, A and B, the null hypothesis is H_o: $P_{AB} = 0.50$ where P_{AB} is the probability that item A is chosen over item B. The alternate is H_1: $P_{AB} = 0.50$.

(*b*) Examples of Use—

(1) A preference test was run with 50 respondents; 34 preferred Sample A and 16 preferred Sample B. Table 1 shows that 33 choices are needed for statistical significance at the 5% risk level with a sample size of 50.

(2) A small-scale test was run to determine whether two samples differed in degree of saltiness. Out of 16 subjects, 12 chose sample A and 4 chose sample B. Because the critical value is 12 at the 10% risk level, sample A is declared to be saltier than sample B at the 90% level of confidence.

(*c*) When the number of judgments exceeds the range of Table 1 use the *t*-test for percentages or the *z*-score.

2. Table 2—Significance of Results in Duo-Trio or One Sided Paired Comparison Situations

(*a*) Table 2 is for use in situations where the choice of only one of the samples will fulfill the conditions of the experiment. It gives the number of correct identifications (critical values) for the 50% chance probability at alpha risk levels of 0.10, 0.05, 0.01, and 0.001. For two samples, A and B, the null hypothesis is H_o: $P_{AB} = 0.50$ where P_{AB} is the probability that item A is chosen over item B. The alternate is H_1: $P_{AB} > 0.50$. This table can also be used for paired difference tests and the duo-trio test.

(*b*) Examples of Use—A duo-trio was run with 20 subjects. There were 16 correct identifications. Enter Table 2 at 20 in the first column and note that the 16 correct is exactly what is required for significance at the 1% level.

(*c*) When the number of judgments exceeds the range of the table, use the *t*-test for percentages.

3. Tables 3a, 3b, and 3c—Critical Values and Power Tables for the Triangle Test

Table 3 is divided into three subtables according to the level of significance being used in the study. Table 3*a* contains entries for the $\alpha = 0.10$ level of significance. Table 3*b* contains entries for the $\alpha = 0.05$ level of significance. Table 3*c* contains entries for the $\alpha = 0.01$ level of significance.

TABLE 3a—*Critical values and power of the triangle test for* α = 0.10.

Column 1 = Sample size.
Column 2 = Critical value (c), the minimum number of correct responses required to conclude that a perceivable difference exists at the α = 0.1 level of significance.
Column 3 to 9 = Power (1 − β), the probability of concluding that a perceivable difference exists when the true probability of correct response is P_D.

		P_D						
n	c	0.40	0.45	0.50	0.55	0.60	0.65	0.70
6	5	0.04	0.07	0.11	0.16	0.23	0.32	0.42
8	5	0.17	0.26	0.36	0.48	0.59	0.71	0.81
10	6	0.17	0.26	0.38	0.50	0.63	0.75	0.85
12	7	0.16	0.26	0.39	0.53	0.67	0.79	0.88
15	8	0.21	0.35	0.50	0.65	0.79	0.89	0.95
20	10	0.24	0.41	0.59	0.75	0.87	0.95	0.98
25	12	0.27	0.46	0.65	0.82	0.92	0.97	0.99
30	14	0.29	0.50	0.71	0.86	0.95	0.99	1.00
35	16	0.30	0.53	0.75	0.90	0.97	0.99	1.00
40	18	0.31	0.56	0.79	0.92	0.98	1.00	1.00
45	20	0.32	0.59	0.81	0.94	0.99	1.00	1.00
50	22	0.33	0.61	0.84	0.96	0.99	1.00	1.00
55	24	0.34	0.63	0.86	0.97	1.00	1.00	1.00
60	26	0.34	0.65	0.88	0.97	1.00	1.00	1.00
65	28	0.35	0.67	0.89	0.98	1.00	1.00	1.00
70	29	0.45	0.76	0.94	0.99	1.00	1.00	1.00
75	31	0.45	0.77	0.95	0.99	1.00	1.00	1.00
80	33	0.45	0.78	0.95	1.00	1.00	1.00	1.00
85	35	0.45	0.79	0.96	1.00	1.00	1.00	1.00
90	37	0.45	0.80	0.96	1.00	1.00	1.00	1.00
95	39	0.46	0.81	0.97	1.00	1.00	1.00	1.00
100	40	0.54	0.87	0.98	1.00	1.00	1.00	1.00

(a) Sample Size, n—The first column of Tables 3a, 3b, and 3c contains the values for sample size, *n*. Most often, the sample size is the number of respondents who participate in the study. However, in same studies the sample size is the number of triangles presented to a single respondent when, for example, the purpose of the study is to measure the respondent's ability to discriminate between two samples, A and B.

(b) Critical Values, c—The second column in Tables 3a, 3b, and 3c contains the critical value, *c*, for a triangle test with sample size *n* and significance level α. The critical value is the minimum number of correct selections required to declare that the two samples in the study are distinguishable at the level of significance being used.

For example, suppose a sensory analyst is running a triangle test with *n* = 30 respondents at the α = 0.05 level of significance. Table 3b indicates that c = 15 or more correct responses are required to declare that a significant (that is, perceivable) difference exists between the two samples in the study. If fewer

TABLE 3b—*Critical values and power of the triangle test for* α = 0.05.

Column 1 = Sample size.
Column 2 = Critical value (c), the minimum number of correct responses required to conclude that a perceivable difference exists at the α = 0.05 level of significance.
Column 3 to 9 = Power (1 − β), the probability of concluding that a perceivable difference exists when the true probability of correct response is P_D.

n	c	P_D						
		0.40	0.45	0.50	0.55	0.60	0.65	0.70
6	5	0.04	0.07	0.11	0.16	0.23	0.32	0.42
8	6	0.05	0.09	0.14	0.22	0.32	0.43	0.55
10	7	0.05	0.10	0.17	0.27	0.38	0.51	0.65
12	8	0.06	0.11	0.19	0.30	0.44	0.58	0.72
15	9	0.10	0.18	0.30	0.45	0.61	0.75	0.87
20	11	0.13	0.25	0.41	0.59	0.76	0.88	0.95
25	13	0.15	0.31	0.50	0.69	0.85	0.94	0.98
30	15	0.18	0.36	0.57	0.77	0.90	0.97	0.99
35	17	0.19	0.40	0.63	0.83	0.94	0.98	1.00
40	19	0.21	0.43	0.68	0.87	0.96	0.99	1.00
45	21	0.22	0.47	0.72	0.90	0.97	1.00	1.00
50	23	0.23	0.50	0.76	0.92	0.98	1.00	1.00
55	25	0.24	0.53	0.79	0.94	0.99	1.00	1.00
60	27	0.25	0.55	0.82	0.95	0.99	1.00	1.00
65	29	0.26	0.57	0.84	0.96	1.00	1.00	1.00
70	31	0.27	0.59	0.86	0.97	1.00	1.00	1.00
75	33	0.28	0.61	0.88	0.98	1.00	1.00	1.00
80	35	0.28	0.63	0.89	0.98	1.00	1.00	1.00
85	37	0.29	0.65	0.90	0.99	1.00	1.00	1.00
90	38	0.37	0.74	0.94	0.99	1.00	1.00	1.00
95	40	0.37	0.75	0.95	1.00	1.00	1.00	1.00
100	42	0.38	0.76	0.96	1.00	1.00	1.00	1.00

than 15 correct responses occur then the analyst cannot conclude that a perceivable difference exists.

(c) *Power, 1 − β*—The remaining columns in Tables 3a, 3b, and 3c contain entries for the power, (1 − β), of the triangle test. Just as it is possible to incorrectly conclude that a perceivable difference exists when one does not, that is, make a Type I error with probability α; it is also possible to fail to detect a difference when one does exist, that is, make a Type II error with probability β. Rather than focusing on the probability of missing a difference, statistical tests are characterized by how likely they are to detect a difference when one exists. The likelihood of detecting a real difference is called the power of the test (Power = 1 − β). The value of the power of a test is a function of the sample size, n; the level of significance, α; and the size of the difference that actually exists, P_D.

Suppose again that a sensory analyst is conducting a triangle test with n = 30 respondents at the α = 0.05 level of significance. From the fifth column of Table 3b it can be seen that this test has a probability of 1 − β = 0.57 of

TABLE 3c—*Critical values and power of the triangle test for* α = 0.01.

Column 1 = Sample size.
Column 2 = Critical value (*c*), the minimum number of correct responses required to conclude that a perceivable difference exists at the α = 0.01 level of significance.
Column 3 to 9 = Power (1 − β), the probability of concluding that a perceivable difference exists when the true probability of correct response is P_D.

		P_D						
n	*c*	0.40	0.45	0.50	0.55	0.60	0.65	0.70
6	6	0.00	0.01	0.02	0.03	0.05	0.08	0.12
8	7	0.01	0.02	0.04	0.06	0.11	0.17	0.26
10	8	0.01	0.03	0.05	0.10	0.17	0.26	0.38
12	9	0.02	0.04	0.07	0.13	0.23	0.35	0.49
15	10	0.03	0.08	0.15	0.26	0.40	0.56	0.72
20	13	0.02	0.06	0.13	0.25	0.42	0.60	0.77
25	15	0.03	0.10	0.21	0.38	0.59	0.77	0.90
30	17	0.05	0.14	0.29	0.50	0.71	0.87	0.96
35	19	0.06	0.17	0.37	0.60	0.81	0.93	0.98
40	21	0.07	0.21	0.44	0.68	0.87	0.96	0.99
45	24	0.05	0.17	0.38	0.65	0.86	0.96	0.99
50	26	0.06	0.20	0.44	0.72	0.90	0.98	1.00
55	28	0.07	0.23	0.50	0.77	0.93	0.99	1.00
60	30	0.07	0.26	0.55	0.82	0.96	0.99	1.00
65	32	0.08	0.29	0.60	0.86	0.97	1.00	1.00
70	34	0.09	0.31	0.64	0.88	0.98	1.00	1.00
75	36	0.10	0.34	0.68	0.91	0.99	1.00	1.00
80	38	0.11	0.37	0.71	0.93	0.99	1.00	1.00
85	40	0.11	0.39	0.74	0.94	0.99	1.00	1.00
90	42	0.12	0.41	0.77	0.95	1.00	1.00	1.00
95	44	0.13	0.44	0.79	0.96	1.00	1.00	1.00
100	46	0.13	0.46	0.82	0.97	1.00	1.00	1.00

detecting the situation where the real probability of selecting the odd sample is P_D = 0.50 instead of the chance probability for a triangle test of 0.33. Stated in another way, a triangle test conducted with *n* = 30 respondents of the α = 0.05 level of significance will fail to detect the case where P_D = 0.50 forty-three percent of the time (43% = 100(1 − Power) = 100 β).

Examination of the tables reveals that the power of the test increases with increasing sample sizes, with increasing levels of significance, and with increasing values of P_D. In practice, developing a triangle test with a specified level of power requires a compromise among available resources, that is, (*n*), reliability (α), and sensitivity (P_D).

(d) Relationship to "Similarity" Tests—The Type I or alpha error (probability of claiming a difference when none exists) is controlled in the calculation of the critical values for the triangle test for a difference while the Type II or beta error (probability of failing to detect a true difference) is controlled in a triangle test for similarity. The power tables given here can be used to determine the likelihood

TABLE 4—*Values of* t *required for significance at various levels for two-tailed and one-tailed for hypotheses.*[a]

		Level of Significance			
Degrees of Freedom	10%[c]	10%[b] 5%	5% 2.5%	2% 1%	1% 0.5%	0.1% 0.05%
1	3.08	6.31	12.71	31.82	63.66	636.62
2	1.89	2.92	4.3	6.96	9.92	31.6
3	1.64	2.35	3.18	4.54	5.84	12.94
4	1.53	2.13	2.78	3.75	4.6	8.61
5	1.48	2.02	2.57	3.36	4.03	6.86
6	1.44	1.94	2.45	3.14	3.71	5.96
7	1.41	1.9	2.36	3.0	3.5	5.4
8	1.4	1.86	2.31	2.9	3.36	5.04
9	1.38	1.83	2.26	2.82	3.25	4.78
10	1.37	1.81	2.23	2.76	3.17	4.59
11	1.36	1.8	2.2	2.72	3.11	4.44
12	1.36	1.78	2.18	2.68	3.06	4.32
13	1.35	1.77	2.16	2.65	3.01	4.22
14	1.34	1.76	2.14	2.62	2.98	4.14
15	1.34	1.75	2.13	2.6	2.95	4.07
16	1.34	1.75	2.12	2.58	2.92	4.02
17	1.33	1.74	2.11	2.57	2.9	3.96
18	1.33	1.73	2.1	2.55	2.88	3.92
19	1.33	1.73	2.09	2.54	2.86	3.88
20	1.33	1.72	2.09	2.53	2.84	3.85
21	1.32	1.72	2.08	2.52	2.83	3.82
22	1.32	1.72	2.07	2.51	2.82	3.79
23	1.32	1.71	2.07	2.5	2.81	3.77
24	1.32	1.71	2.06	2.49	2.8	3.74
25	1.32	1.71	2.06	2.48	2.79	3.72
26	1.32	1.71	2.06	2.48	2.78	3.71
27	1.31	1.7	2.05	2.47	2.77	3.69
28	1.31	1.7	2.05	2.46	2.76	3.67
29	1.31	1.7	2.04	2.46	2.76	3.66
30	1.31	1.7	2.04	2.46	2.75	3.65
40	1.3	1.68	2.02	2.42	2.7	3.55
60	1.3	1.67	2.0	2.39	2.66	3.46
120	1.29	1.66	1.98	2.36	2.62	3.37
∞ (infinity)	1.28	1.64	1.96	2.33	2.58	3.29

[a]This table is abridged from Table III of Fisher and Yates, Statistical Tables for Biological, Agricultural and Medical Research, 6th ed., Oliver and Boyd, Edinburg, 1863, by permission of the authors and publishers.
[b]Two tailed hypothesis.
[c]One-tailed hypothesis.

that a triangle test with a given number of respondents will detect a difference of a given size, which is equivalent to a similarity test. Alternatively, tables of critical values for a triangle test for similarity are given in Sensory Evaluation Techniques. (See bibliography at the end of the chapter.)

(e) Example of Use of Critical Values—A triangle test was run with 50 subjects. There were 30 correct identifications. Table 5c shows that only 26 correct are needed to conclude a significant difference even at the 1% risk level.

(f) *Example of Use of Power Tables*—Suppose that a sample size for a triangle test is desired that will allow us to conclude with a beta risk of 0.05 (1 − β = 0.95) that A and B are different when the difference P_D is as large as 0.70. We also want to set the risk of rejecting the null hypothesis of equality when it is true at 0.05. Table 3*b* shows that a sample size of 20 triangles is sufficient. The critical value is 11 correct choices.

(g) *Note*—When the number of judgments exceeds the range of the table, use the *t*-test for proportions.

E. The *t*-Test

The *t*-test is one of the most commonly used statistical procedures in determining the significance of the difference between two results. The T-statistic is a ratio of the difference to the standard error of that difference. Another property of the *t*-statistic is that it gives information about the direction of the difference. In some applications this information is quite important to the interpretation of the results. There are tables of the *t*-distribution which give the *t*-values for certain probabilities and degrees of freedom. Table 4 is an example. Some calculators and computer software packages can calculate the exact probability from the T-value and the degrees of freedom. There are many applications of this test. However, there are basically only four forms which are used in the frame of reference of this manual.

1. The Generalized t-Test

The most common method is the general *t*-test for difference between two independent groups of data. The assumptions made about the two data sets are that they have roughly the same variance and that they come from populations with "normal" distributions. There does not need to be the same number of observations in each set. The data from page 82 can be used as an example of the calculations.

Suppose that the two sets of data represent ratings of a sample on a 7-point scale. Set A is from one group of 10 respondents and set B is from a second group of respondents. The question is: did the two groups differ in their average rating of the sample?

	Set A	Set B
Mean rating	4.7	3.7
Variance	1.789	2.233
Standard deviation	1.337	1.494
SEM	0.423	0.472

$$\text{SE of difference} = \sqrt{\frac{1.789 + 2.233}{10}} = \sqrt{\frac{4.022}{10}} = 0.634$$

$$t = \frac{4.7 - 3.7}{0.634} = \frac{1.0}{0.634} = 1.577$$

$$df = (10 - 1) + (10 - 1) = 18$$

From Table 4 it is found that for 18 degrees of freedom a t-value of 2.10 is necessary for significance at the 5% level. Since the calculated t-value of 1.577 is less than 2.10 it can be stated that the averages of the two groups are not significantly different at the 5% level (the null hypothesis is not rejected).

2. The Paired t-Test

The data sets to be examined may sometimes be "paired." That is, each value of the first set is like the same value from the second set in all respects but one. For example, each respondent rates sample A and sample B. Then the only difference in the ratings from any given respondent is the difference between sample A and sample B. This situation allows a simpler calculation using the differences. It also provides a more powerful test of significance because it removes the variation due to differences in scoring level among the respondents. The statistical test is to determine whether the observed average difference is significantly different from zero.

Let us now suppose that the illustrative data set represents the ratings of ten respondents on each of two samples, A and B. Since each respondent tested both samples, the data are paired. The t-statistic is calculated from the difference columns of the illustrative data set as follows:

$$t = \frac{\bar{d}}{\text{SEM}(d)}$$

$$= \frac{1.0}{0.745} = 1.34$$

with $(10 - 1) = 9$ df

From Table 4 it is found that for 9 degrees of freedom a t-value of 2.26 is necessary for significance at the 5% level. Since the calculated t-value of 1.34 is less than 2.26 it can be stated that the average difference is not significantly different from zero at the 5% level (the null hypothesis is not rejected).

It is important to note the difference in the t-value for this test compared to the t-value found previously in the second part of the general t-test. The stipulations for the two tests are different even though the questions are essentially the same. It is possible that one test could show significance but not the other! One must be careful that the conditions for the paired t-test are met otherwise erroneous conclusions could be drawn.

TABLE 5—*Values of chi-square required for significance at various levels.*[a]

Degrees of Freedom	Level of Significance				
	10%	5%	2.5%	1%	0.5%
1	2.71	3.84	5.02	6.63	7.83
2	4.61	5.99	7.38	9.21	10.6
3	6.25	7.81	9.35	11.3	12.8
4	7.78	9.49	11.1	13.3	14.9
5	9.24	11.1	12.8	15.1	16.7
6	10.60	12.6	14.4	16.8	18.5
7	12.0	14.1	16.0	18.5	20.3
8	13.4	15.5	17.5	20.1	22.0
9	14.7	16.9	19.0	21.7	23.6
10	16.0	18.3	20.5	23.2	25.2
11	17.3	19.7	21.9	24.7	26.8
12	18.5	21.0	23.3	26.2	28.3
13	19.8	22.4	24.7	27.7	29.8
14	21.1	23.7	26.1	29.1	31.3
15	22.3	25.0	27.5	30.6	32.8
16	23.5	26.3	28.8	32.0	34.3
17	24.8	27.6	30.2	33.4	35.7
18	26.0	28.9	31.5	34.8	37.2
19	27.2	30.1	32.9	36.2	38.6
20	28.4	31.4	34.2	37.6	40.0
21	29.6	32.7	35.5	38.9	41.4
22	30.8	33.9	36.8	40.3	42.8
23	32.0	35.2	38.1	41.6	44.2
24	33.2	36.4	39.4	43.0	45.6
25	34.4	37.7	40.6	44.3	46.5
26	35.6	38.9	41.9	45.6	48.3
27	36.7	40.1	43.2	47.0	49.6
28	37.9	41.3	44.5	48.3	51.0
29	39.1	42.6	45.7	49.6	52.3
30	40.3	43.8	47.0	50.9	53.7

[a]Abridged with permission of the publisher from a table that originally appeared in an article by Thompson, Catherine M., *Biometrika*, Vol. 32, pp. 188 and 189.

3. The t-Test for Proportions

The *t*-test can also be used to determine the significance of differences between proportions. The only new calculation is the estimate of the standard error of a proportion. It is calculated from

$$SE = \sqrt{\frac{p \cdot q}{n}}$$

where

p = proportion,
$q = 1 - p$, and
n = total number of observations in the proportion.

The standard error of the difference of two proportions is given by

$$SE_{AB} = \sqrt{SE_A^2 + SE_B^2}$$

The t-test for proportions is most often used to determine the significance of the difference between an experimentally obtained proportion and a fixed proportion such as the 50:50 theoretical chance proportion in a paired comparison. It may also be used to determine the significance of the difference between two experimentally obtained proportions.

To illustrate the first use, suppose that a preference test was run between sample A and sample B by 120 judges; 72 preferred A and 48 preferred B. The chance proportion is 0.50, and the standard error of the chance proportion is

$$SE = \sqrt{\frac{0.50 \cdot 0.50}{120}}$$

$$= \frac{0.50}{10.945} = 0.046$$

The observed proportion is

$$\frac{72}{120} = 0.600$$

$$t = \frac{0.600 - 0.500}{0.046} = \frac{0.100}{0.046} = 2.17$$

$$df = 120$$

From Table 4 the t-value for 5% significance and 120 df is 1.98. The calculated value is greater than the tabled value and the proportion is significantly different from that expected by chance at the 5% level (the null hypothesis is rejected). The t-value at 1% is 2.62. The calculated value is less than that tabled value so the null hypothesis cannot be rejected at the 1% level. Therefore, the significance of the difference lies between 5 and 1%. In this case the degrees of freedom were equal to the maximum table degrees of freedom. However, if the actual degrees of freedom are between 121 and 159 the t-value for 120 degrees of freedom may be used without introducing an unacceptable error. If the actual degrees of freedom are 160 or more the table entries for infinite degrees of freedom should be used.

To illustrate the second use, suppose that in a second group of 100 judges 58 chose sample A and 42 chose sample B. Did the two groups show a significant difference in preference?

$$SE_1 = \sqrt{\frac{0.595 \cdot 0.0405}{121}} = \sqrt{\frac{0.2410}{121}} = 0.0446$$

$$SE_2 = \sqrt{\frac{0.580 \cdot 0.420}{100}} = \sqrt{\frac{0.2436}{100}} = 0.0494$$

$$SE_{(A-B)} = \sqrt{0.001989 + 0.002440} = \sqrt{0.004429} = 0.0666$$

$$t = \frac{0.595 - 0.580}{0.0666} = \frac{0.015}{0.0666} = 0.227$$

The calculated t-value is less than 1.00 and is less than any t-value in Table 4; therefore, there is no significant difference between the proportions from the two groups of judges.

4. The t-Test of an Average Against a Fixed Value

In some cases one may wish to compare the average of a set of results against some fixed value such as a target or specification. The calculations are similar to those for the generalized t-test

$$t = \frac{(x - k)}{(s/\sqrt{n})}$$

where

x = mean of the test data set,
k = fixed value,
s = standard deviation of the test data set, and
n = number of values in the test data set.

For example, suppose that a product is reformulated but must retain a rating of 7.0 on some attribute scale. A panel of 40 judges gives a trial product an average rating of 6.3 with a standard deviation of 0.9. Is this trial product acceptably close to the target? From this information the t-value, with 39 degrees of freedom, is

$$t = \frac{(6.3 - 7.0)}{(0.9/\sqrt{40})} = \frac{-0.7}{0.142} = -4.92$$

This t-value is greater than any value for either 30 or 40 degrees of freedom in Table 4. It can be stated that the null hypothesis is rejected, and the test product differs significantly from the target. The minus sign of the t-value shows that the test results were lower than the target.

F. Chi-Square Test

1. This is a method to determine whether the distribution of observed frequencies of a categorical variable (either nominal or ordinal) differs significantly from the distribution of frequencies which are expected according to some hypothesis. The chi-square test is to categorical data what t-tests and analysis of variance are to interval data.

2. Critical values (Table 5) of the distribution of chi-square are published in tables which appear in most statistical texts. They show the values which are required for statistical significance at various significance levels and for various degrees of freedom.

3. It is important that the hypothesis be one which is meaningful in regard to the particular experiment. In most cases this will be obvious. For example, when using the null hypothesis that there is no real difference between samples in regard to the characteristic measured, the responses should be equally divided among the categories as in

			Category		
	1	2	3	4	Total
Observed	O_1	O_2	O_3	O_4	n
Expected	$n/4$	$n/4$	$n/4$	$n/4$	

Another situation is where a test has been run in two (or more) situations or with two (or more) different groups of people. The null hypothesis in this case is that the multiple sets of observed frequencies all arise from the same distribution. Here one "averages" the multiple frequencies in each category to obtain the expected frequency. For example, when equal numbers of observations are collected from each of two groups, the expected frequencies are the simple arithmetic means of the observed frequencies, as shown next. When unequal numbers of observations are collected from each group a more complicated calculation is used to obtain the expected frequencies (see Number 7).

		Category			
Group	1	2	3	4	Total
1	O_{11}	O_{12}	O_{13}	O_{14}	n
2	O_{21}	O_{22}	O_{23}	O_{24}	n
Expected	$\dfrac{O_{11} + O_{21}}{2n}$	$\dfrac{O_{12} + O_{22}}{2n}$	$\dfrac{O_{13} + O_{23}}{2n}$	$\dfrac{O_{14} + O_{24}}{2n}$	$2n$

4. The formula for chi-square is

$$X^2 = \sum \frac{(O - E)^2}{E}$$

where

O = frequency observed, and
E = frequency expected.

The expected frequency in each term of the chi-square should be five or more ($E \geq 5$) to ensure the accuracy of the p-values obtained in tests of hypotheses. For situations in which some of the expected values are less than 5 it is sometimes possible to collapse some of the categories to obtain larger expected values.

5. The calculated chi-square value is interpreted by reference to published tables (see Table 5) which show the values to be expected at selected significance levels according to degrees of freedom. Calculated values larger than those in the table are significant. Alternatively, computer programs that compute chi-square tests and their associated p-values are widely available. If the p-value from a computer program is smaller than the pre-selected significance level (for example, $\alpha \doteq 0.05$) then the test is significant.

6. Example of application to preference data:

Null Hypothesis: All samples are equally preferred.
Observed number of choices: A = 28, B = 12.
Expected number of choices: A = 20, B = 20.
Degrees of freedom: (No. of categories − 1) = 1

$$X^2 = \frac{(28 - 20)^2}{20} + \frac{(12 - 20)^2}{20} = 3.2 + 3.2 = 6.4$$

Entering the chi-square table with one degree of freedom, we find that 6.4 is to be expected by chance only about 1% of the time; hence, the result is significant at approximately that level. (This example is the categorical-data analog to the single sample t-test used for interval data.)

7. Example of application to a multiple location test (with unequal numbers of observations at each site).

Null Hypothesis: The distributions of frequencies among categories A, B, and C are the same at both test locations.

Observed results:

| Location | Category | | | Total |
	A	B	C	
1	12	24	44	80
2	25	40	55	120
Total	37	64	99	200

Expected results:

| Location | Category | | | Total |
	A	B	C	
1	14.8	25.6	39.6	80
2	22.2	38.4	59.4	120
Total	37	64	99	200

where, for example, $E_{1A} = (80)(37)/200 = 14.8$

Degrees of freedom: (No. of rows $-$ 1)(No. of columns $-$ 1) = 2

$$X^2 = 0.530 + 0.100 + 0.489 + 0.353 + 0.067 + 0.326 = 1.864$$

Entering the chi-square table with two degrees of freedom, we find that 1.864 is much smaller than the smallest critical value in the Table 5 (that is, 4.61 for the 10% significance level). Therefore, we conclude that the results do not provide sufficient basis to conclude that the distributions differ between the two locations. (This example is the categorical-data analog to the two-sample t-test used for interval data.)

8. Example of application to paired, categorical data (McNemar test):

Test design: Each respondent receives two pairs of samples—a matched pair, either AA or BB, and an unmatched pair, AB or BA. For each pair the respondents indicate whether the samples are the same or different.

Null hypothesis: Samples A and B are not perceptibly different.

Observed results:

		Received AA or BB and Responded	
		Same	Different
Received AB or BA	Same	a = 7	b = 28
Responded	Different	c = 47	d = 18

Frequencies a and d represent "ties" and contribute no information for determining if the samples are different. Only frequencies b and c are used to calculate the test statistic.

$$X^2 = (b - c)2/(b + c) = (28 - 47)2/(28 + 47) = 4.81$$

Degrees of freedom: 1

The value 4.81 is greater than the 5% significance value of a X^2 with one degree of freedom, so it is concluded that the two samples are perceptibly different. If two samples are compared using a categorical scale with more than two categories, then a Stuart-Maxwell test should be used. (Both the McNemar and the Stuart-Maxwell tests are categorical-data analogs to the paired t-test used for interval data.)

9. Example of application of chi-square to rank order data: (Seven samples have been ranked for preference by 14 subjects.)

				Sample			
Subject	A	B	C	D	E	F	G
1	1	3	2	6	5	4	7
2	1	2	3	4	6	5	7
4	1	4	2	3	7	5	6
5	1	3	2	4	5	6	7
6	1	2	3	6	5	4	7
7	2	1	3	5	4	7	6
9	3	1	2	6	4	5	7
10	1	4	2	3	5	6	7
11	1	3	2	5	4	6	7
12	1	2	3	5	4	6	7
13	1	3	4	2	7	6	5
14	2	3	4	5	1	7	6
Rank Total	18	36	39	61	68	77	93

$$X^2 = \left(\frac{12}{np(p + 1)}\right) \sum (Ri)^2 - 3n(p + 1)$$

where

n = number of subjects,
p = number of samples (and number of ranks),
R_i = rank sum for sample 1, and
$p + 1$ = degrees of freedom.

$$X^2 = \frac{12}{(14)(7)(8)} \, 26\,064 - 3(14)(8) = 62.92$$

The chi-square table (Table 5) shows that for six degrees of freedom a value as high as 62.9 will occur by chance only 1% of the time. Therefore, differences among the samples have been established at less than the 1% risk level.

G. Analysis of Variance

1. Analysis of Variance

This is a method used to test for significant differences in treatment or product means and to estimate variance components. The analysis depends upon the experimental design and can be very complex going far beyond any exposition that might be attempted within the scope of this manual. It is recommended to consult with a statistician to make sure that the design meets the needs. User friendly software to do analysis of variance can be obtained readily for both the main frame and the personal computer. Thus, detailed calculations are not provided here.

2. Basic Ideas of Analysis of Variance

(*a.*) The total amount of variation that exists within a distribution of scores (values, measures) can be split into components of variance such as product-type-to-product-type variation, subject to subject variation, and within-subject variation. Some components represent planned differences called fixed effects (treatments, factors); others are random effects such as measurement error.

(*b.*) If the variance among fixed effects exceeds the variation within such effects, the fixed effects are said to be statistically different. The F-distribution is used to compare the ratio of the fixed effects variance to the random variance, called error. In an analysis of variance table the mean square values are used to compare the variances (see the discussion in 3*b*). The critical values for the *F*-distribution are given in Tables 6*a*, *b*, and *c* for 10, 5, and 1% risk levels, respectively. If the calculated *F*-value exceeds the critical value, one or more treatment means are statistically different. The errors are assumed to be independently and normally distributed. If they are not normally distributed, a transformation of the data will often make them so. The most common transformations are the logarithm and the square root.

3. Example: 2 Factor Experiment

(*a*) Three judges have scored five samples (1, 2, 3, 4, and 5) each of which was prepared twice. The data appear in the following:

Respondent	Sample									
	1	1	2	2	3	3	4	4	5	5
A	5	4	4.5	4	1	1	5.5	6	6	5.5
B	4	4.5	4	5	1	1	5.5	6.5	6.5	6
C	4.5	4	4.5	4	1	1	6.5	6	5	5.5

The average values are:

Respondents			
A	B	C	
4.25	4.4	4.2	LSD = 0.4

Samples				
1	2	3	4	5
4.3	4.3	1.0	6.0	5.8	LSD = 0.5

Analysis of variance can be used to assess the significance of observed differences among samples and among subjects. In this example, the multiple preparations are considered to be random effects.

NOTE: LSD is the least significant difference between means.

TABLE 6a—Values of F-ratio significant at the 10% level.[a]

n_2[c] \ n_1[b]	1	2	3	4	5	6	7	8	9	10	12	15	20	24	30	40	60	120	∞
1	39.86	49.50	53.59	55.83	57.24	58.20	58.91	59.44	59.86	60.19	60.71	61.22	61.74	62.00	62.26	62.53	62.79	63.06	63.33
2	8.53	9.00	9.16	9.24	9.29	9.33	9.35	9.37	9.38	9.39	9.41	9.42	9.44	9.45	9.46	9.47	9.47	9.48	9.49
3	5.54	5.46	5.39	5.34	5.31	5.28	5.27	5.25	5.24	5.23	5.22	5.20	5.18	5.18	5.17	5.16	5.15	5.14	5.13
4	4.54	4.32	4.19	4.11	4.05	4.01	3.98	3.95	3.94	3.92	3.90	3.87	3.84	3.83	3.82	3.80	3.79	3.78	3.76
5	4.06	3.78	3.62	3.52	3.45	3.40	3.37	3.34	3.32	3.30	3.27	3.24	3.21	3.19	3.17	3.16	3.14	3.12	3.10
6	3.78	3.46	3.29	3.18	3.11	3.05	3.01	2.98	2.96	2.94	2.90	2.87	2.84	2.82	2.80	2.78	2.76	2.74	2.72
7	3.59	3.26	3.07	2.96	2.88	2.83	2.78	2.75	2.72	2.70	2.67	2.63	2.59	2.58	2.56	2.54	2.51	2.49	2.47
8	3.46	3.11	2.92	2.81	2.73	2.67	2.62	2.59	2.56	2.54	2.50	2.46	2.42	2.40	2.38	2.36	2.34	2.32	2.29
9	3.36	3.01	2.81	2.69	2.61	2.55	2.51	2.47	2.44	2.42	2.38	2.34	2.30	2.28	2.25	2.23	2.21	2.18	2.16
10	3.29	2.92	2.73	2.61	2.52	2.46	2.41	2.38	2.35	2.32	2.28	2.24	2.20	2.18	2.16	2.13	2.11	2.08	2.06
11	3.23	2.86	2.66	2.54	2.45	2.39	2.34	2.30	2.27	2.25	2.21	2.17	2.12	2.10	2.08	2.05	2.03	2.00	1.97
12	3.18	2.81	2.61	2.48	2.39	2.33	2.28	2.24	2.21	2.19	2.15	2.10	2.06	2.04	2.01	1.99	1.96	1.93	1.90
13	3.14	2.76	2.56	2.43	2.35	2.28	2.23	2.20	2.16	2.14	2.10	2.05	2.01	1.98	1.96	1.93	1.90	1.88	1.85
14	3.10	2.73	2.52	2.39	2.31	2.24	2.19	2.15	2.12	2.10	2.05	2.01	1.96	1.94	1.91	1.89	1.86	1.83	1.80
15	3.07	2.70	2.49	2.36	2.27	2.21	2.16	2.12	2.09	2.06	2.02	1.97	1.92	1.90	1.87	1.85	1.82	1.79	1.76
16	3.05	2.67	2.46	2.33	2.24	2.18	2.13	2.09	2.06	2.03	1.99	1.94	1.89	1.87	1.84	1.81	1.78	1.75	1.72
17	3.03	2.64	2.44	2.31	2.22	2.15	2.10	2.06	2.03	2.00	1.96	1.91	1.86	1.84	1.81	1.78	1.75	1.72	1.69
18	3.01	2.62	2.42	2.29	2.20	2.13	2.08	2.04	2.00	1.98	1.93	1.89	1.84	1.81	1.78	1.75	1.72	1.69	1.66
19	2.99	2.61	2.40	2.27	2.18	2.11	2.06	2.02	1.98	1.96	1.91	1.86	1.81	1.79	1.76	1.73	1.70	1.67	1.63
20	2.97	2.59	2.38	2.25	2.16	2.09	2.04	2.00	1.96	1.94	1.89	1.84	1.79	1.77	1.74	1.71	1.68	1.64	1.61
21	2.96	2.57	2.36	2.23	2.14	2.08	2.02	1.98	1.95	1.92	1.87	1.83	1.78	1.75	1.72	1.69	1.66	1.62	1.59
22	2.95	2.56	2.35	2.22	2.13	2.06	2.01	1.97	1.93	1.90	1.86	1.81	1.76	1.73	1.70	1.67	1.64	1.60	1.57
23	2.94	2.55	2.34	2.21	2.11	2.05	1.99	1.95	1.92	1.89	1.84	1.80	1.74	1.72	1.69	1.66	1.62	1.59	1.55
24	2.93	2.54	2.33	2.19	2.10	2.04	1.98	1.94	1.91	1.88	1.83	1.78	1.73	1.70	1.67	1.64	1.61	1.57	1.53
25	2.92	2.53	2.32	2.18	2.09	2.02	1.97	1.93	1.89	1.87	1.82	1.77	1.72	1.69	1.66	1.63	1.59	1.56	1.52
26	2.91	2.52	2.31	2.17	2.08	2.01	1.96	1.92	1.88	1.86	1.81	1.76	1.71	1.68	1.65	1.61	1.58	1.54	1.50
27	2.90	2.51	2.30	2.17	2.07	2.00	1.95	1.91	1.87	1.85	1.80	1.75	1.70	1.67	1.64	1.60	1.57	1.53	1.49
28	2.89	2.50	2.29	2.16	2.06	2.00	1.94	1.90	1.87	1.84	1.79	1.74	1.69	1.66	1.63	1.59	1.56	1.52	1.48
29	2.89	2.50	2.28	2.15	2.06	1.99	1.93	1.89	1.86	1.83	1.78	1.73	1.68	1.65	1.62	1.58	1.55	1.51	1.47
30	2.88	2.49	2.28	2.14	2.05	1.98	1.93	1.88	1.85	1.82	1.77	1.72	1.67	1.64	1.61	1.57	1.54	1.50	1.46
40	2.84	2.44	2.23	2.09	2.00	1.93	1.87	1.83	1.79	1.76	1.71	1.66	1.61	1.57	1.54	1.51	1.47	1.42	1.38
60	2.79	2.39	2.18	2.04	1.95	1.87	1.82	1.77	1.74	1.71	1.66	1.60	1.54	1.51	1.48	1.44	1.40	1.35	1.29
120	2.75	2.35	2.13	1.99	1.90	1.82	1.77	1.72	1.68	1.65	1.60	1.55	1.48	1.45	1.41	1.37	1.32	1.26	1.19
∞	2.71	2.30	2.08	1.94	1.85	1.77	1.72	1.67	1.63	1.60	1.55	1.49	1.42	1.38	1.34	1.30	1.24	1.17	1.00

[a]Adapted with permission from *Biometrika Tables for Statisticians*, 2nd ed., Vol. 1, Pearson, E. S. and Hartly, H. O., Eds., Cambridge University Press, New York, 1958.

[b]n_1 = degrees of freedom for numerator.

TABLE 6b—Values of F-ratio significant at the 5% level.[a]

n_2[c] \ n_1[b]	1	2	3	4	5	6	7	8	9	10	12	15	20	24	30	40	60	120	∞
1	161.40	199.50	215.70	224.60	230.20	234.00	236.80	238.90	240.50	241.90	243.90	245.90	248.00	249.10	250.10	251.10	252.20	253.30	254.3
2	18.51	19.00	19.16	19.25	19.30	19.33	19.35	19.37	19.38	19.40	19.41	19.43	19.45	19.45	19.46	19.47	19.48	19.49	19.50
3	10.13	9.55	9.28	9.12	9.01	8.94	8.89	8.85	8.81	8.79	8.74	8.70	8.66	8.64	8.62	8.59	8.57	8.55	8.53
4	7.71	6.94	6.59	6.39	6.26	6.16	6.09	6.04	6.00	5.96	5.91	5.86	5.80	5.77	5.75	5.72	5.69	5.66	5.63
5	6.61	5.79	5.41	5.19	5.05	4.95	4.88	4.82	4.77	4.74	4.68	4.62	4.56	4.53	4.50	4.46	4.43	4.40	4.36
6	5.99	5.14	4.76	4.53	4.39	4.28	4.21	4.15	4.10	4.06	4.00	3.94	3.87	3.84	3.81	3.77	3.74	3.70	3.67
7	5.59	4.74	4.35	4.12	3.97	3.87	3.79	3.73	3.68	3.64	3.57	3.51	3.44	3.41	3.38	3.34	3.30	3.27	3.23
8	5.32	4.46	4.07	3.84	3.69	3.58	3.50	3.44	3.39	3.35	3.28	3.22	3.15	3.12	3.08	3.04	3.01	2.97	2.93
9	5.12	4.26	3.86	3.63	3.48	3.37	3.29	3.23	3.18	3.14	3.07	3.01	2.94	2.90	2.86	2.83	2.79	2.75	2.71
10	4.96	4.10	3.71	3.48	3.33	3.22	3.14	3.07	3.02	2.98	2.91	2.85	2.77	2.74	2.70	2.66	2.62	2.58	2.54
11	4.84	3.98	3.59	3.36	3.20	3.09	3.01	2.95	2.90	2.85	2.79	2.72	2.65	2.61	2.57	2.53	2.49	2.45	2.40
12	4.75	3.89	3.49	3.26	3.11	3.00	2.91	2.85	2.80	2.75	2.69	2.62	2.54	2.51	2.47	2.43	2.38	2.34	2.30
13	4.67	3.81	3.41	3.18	3.03	2.92	2.83	2.77	2.71	2.67	2.60	2.53	2.46	2.42	2.38	2.34	2.30	2.25	2.21
14	4.60	3.74	3.34	3.11	2.96	2.85	2.76	2.70	2.65	2.60	2.53	2.46	2.39	2.35	2.31	2.27	2.22	2.18	2.13
15	4.54	3.68	3.29	3.06	2.90	2.79	2.71	2.64	2.59	2.54	2.48	2.40	2.33	2.29	2.25	2.20	2.16	2.11	2.07
16	4.49	3.63	3.24	3.01	2.85	2.74	2.66	2.59	2.54	2.49	2.42	2.35	2.28	2.24	2.19	2.15	2.11	2.06	2.01
17	4.45	3.59	3.20	2.96	2.81	2.70	2.61	2.55	2.49	2.45	2.38	2.31	2.23	2.19	2.15	2.10	2.06	2.01	1.96
18	4.41	3.55	3.16	2.93	2.77	2.66	2.58	2.51	2.46	2.41	2.34	2.27	2.19	2.15	2.11	2.06	2.02	1.97	1.92
19	4.38	3.52	3.13	2.90	2.74	2.63	2.54	2.48	2.42	2.38	2.31	2.23	2.16	2.11	2.07	2.03	1.98	1.93	1.88
20	4.35	3.49	3.10	2.87	2.71	2.60	2.51	2.45	2.39	2.35	2.28	2.20	2.12	2.08	2.04	1.99	1.95	1.90	1.84
21	4.32	3.47	3.07	2.84	2.68	2.57	2.49	2.42	2.37	2.32	2.25	2.18	2.10	2.05	2.01	1.96	1.92	1.87	1.81
22	4.30	3.44	3.05	2.82	2.66	2.55	2.46	2.40	2.34	2.30	2.23	2.15	2.07	2.03	1.98	1.94	1.89	1.84	1.78
23	4.28	3.42	3.03	2.80	2.64	2.53	2.44	2.37	2.32	2.27	2.20	2.13	2.05	2.01	1.96	1.91	1.86	1.81	1.76
24	4.26	3.40	3.01	2.78	2.62	2.51	2.42	2.36	2.30	2.25	2.18	2.11	2.03	1.98	1.94	1.89	1.84	1.79	1.73
25	4.24	3.39	2.99	2.76	2.60	2.49	2.40	2.34	2.28	2.24	2.16	2.09	2.01	1.96	1.92	1.87	1.82	1.77	1.71
26	4.23	3.37	2.98	2.74	2.59	2.47	2.39	2.32	2.27	2.22	2.15	2.07	1.99	1.95	1.90	1.85	1.80	1.75	1.69
27	4.21	3.35	2.96	2.73	2.57	2.46	2.37	2.31	2.25	2.20	2.13	2.06	1.97	1.93	1.88	1.84	1.79	1.73	1.67
28	4.20	3.34	2.95	2.71	2.56	2.45	2.36	2.29	2.24	2.19	2.12	2.04	1.96	1.91	1.87	1.82	1.77	1.71	1.65
29	4.18	3.33	2.93	2.70	2.55	2.43	2.35	2.28	2.22	2.18	2.10	2.03	1.94	1.90	1.85	1.81	1.75	1.70	1.64
30	4.17	3.32	2.92	2.69	2.53	2.42	2.33	2.27	2.21	2.16	2.09	2.01	1.93	1.89	1.84	1.79	1.74	1.68	1.62
40	4.08	3.23	2.84	2.61	2.45	2.34	2.25	2.18	2.12	2.08	2.00	1.92	1.84	1.79	1.74	1.69	1.64	1.58	1.51
60	4.00	3.15	2.76	2.53	2.37	2.25	2.17	2.10	2.04	1.99	1.92	1.84	1.75	1.70	1.65	1.59	1.53	1.47	1.39
120	3.92	3.07	2.68	2.45	2.29	2.17	2.09	2.02	1.96	1.91	1.83	1.75	1.66	1.61	1.55	1.50	1.43	1.35	1.25
∞	3.84	3.00	2.60	2.37	2.21	2.10	2.01	1.94	1.88	1.83	1.75	1.67	1.57	1.52	1.46	1.39	1.32	1.22	1.00

[a]Adapted with permission from *Biometrika Tables for Statisticians*, 2nd ed., Vol. 1, Pearson, E. S. and Hartly, H. O., Eds., Cambridge University Press, New York, 1958.
[b]n_1 = degrees of freedom for numerator.
[c]n_2 = degrees of freedom for denominator.

TABLE 6c—Values of F-ratio significant at the 1% level.[a]

n_2[c]	\ n_1[b] 1	2	3	4	5	6	7	8	9	10	12	15	20	24	30	40	60	120	8
1	4052.0	4999.5	5403.0	5625.0	5764.0	5859.0	5928.0	5982.0	6022.0	6056.0	6106.0	6157.0	6209.0	6235.0	6261.0	6287.0	6313.0	6339.0	6366.0
2	98.50	99.00	99.17	99.25	99.30	99.33	99.36	99.37	99.39	99.40	99.42	99.43	99.45	99.46	99.47	99.47	99.48	99.49	99.50
3	34.12	30.82	29.46	28.71	28.24	27.91	27.67	27.49	27.35	27.23	27.05	26.87	26.69	26.60	26.50	26.41	26.32	26.22	26.13
4	21.20	18.00	16.69	15.98	15.52	15.21	14.98	14.80	14.66	14.55	14.37	14.20	14.02	13.93	13.84	13.75	13.65	13.56	13.46
5	16.26	13.27	12.06	11.39	10.97	10.67	10.46	10.29	10.16	10.05	9.89	9.72	9.55	9.47	9.38	9.29	9.20	9.11	9.02
6	13.75	10.92	9.78	9.15	8.75	8.47	8.26	8.10	7.98	7.87	7.72	7.56	7.40	7.31	7.23	7.14	7.06	6.97	6.88
7	12.25	9.55	8.45	7.85	7.46	7.19	6.99	6.84	6.72	6.62	6.47	6.31	6.16	6.07	5.99	5.91	5.82	5.74	5.65
8	11.26	8.65	7.59	7.01	6.63	6.37	6.18	6.03	5.91	5.81	5.67	5.52	5.36	5.28	5.20	5.12	5.03	4.95	4.86
9	10.56	8.02	6.99	6.42	6.06	5.80	5.61	5.47	5.35	5.26	5.11	4.96	4.81	4.73	4.65	4.57	4.48	4.40	4.31
10	10.04	7.56	6.55	5.99	5.64	5.39	5.20	5.06	4.94	4.85	4.71	4.56	4.41	4.33	4.25	4.17	4.08	4.00	3.91
11	9.65	7.21	6.22	5.67	5.32	5.07	4.89	4.74	4.63	4.54	4.40	4.25	4.10	4.02	3.94	3.86	3.78	3.69	3.60
12	9.33	6.93	5.95	5.41	5.06	4.82	4.64	4.50	4.39	4.30	4.16	4.01	3.86	3.78	3.70	3.62	3.54	3.45	3.36
13	9.07	6.70	5.74	5.21	4.86	4.62	4.44	4.30	4.19	4.10	3.96	3.82	3.66	3.59	3.51	3.43	3.34	3.25	3.17
14	8.86	6.51	5.56	5.04	4.69	4.46	4.28	4.14	4.03	3.94	3.80	3.66	3.51	3.43	3.35	3.27	3.18	3.09	3.00
15	8.68	6.36	5.42	4.89	4.56	4.32	4.14	4.00	3.89	3.80	3.67	3.52	3.37	3.29	3.21	3.13	3.05	2.96	2.87
16	8.53	6.23	5.29	4.77	4.44	4.20	4.03	3.89	3.78	3.69	3.55	3.41	3.26	3.18	3.10	3.02	2.93	2.84	2.75
17	8.40	6.11	5.18	4.67	4.34	4.10	3.93	3.79	3.68	3.59	3.46	3.31	3.16	3.08	3.00	2.92	2.83	2.75	2.65
18	8.29	6.01	5.09	4.58	4.25	4.01	3.84	3.71	3.60	3.51	3.37	3.23	3.08	3.00	2.92	2.84	2.75	2.66	2.57
19	8.18	5.93	5.01	4.50	4.17	3.94	3.77	3.63	3.52	3.43	3.30	3.15	3.00	2.92	2.84	2.76	2.67	2.58	2.49
20	8.10	5.85	4.94	4.43	4.10	3.87	3.70	3.56	3.46	3.37	3.23	3.09	2.94	2.86	2.78	2.69	2.61	2.52	2.42
21	8.02	5.78	4.87	4.37	4.04	3.81	3.64	3.51	3.40	3.31	3.17	3.03	2.88	2.80	2.72	2.64	2.55	2.46	2.36
22	7.95	5.72	4.82	4.31	3.99	3.76	3.59	3.45	3.35	3.26	3.12	2.98	2.83	2.75	2.67	2.58	2.50	2.40	2.31
23	7.88	5.66	4.76	4.26	3.94	3.71	3.54	3.41	3.30	3.21	3.07	2.93	2.78	2.70	2.62	2.54	2.45	2.35	2.26
24	7.82	5.61	4.72	4.22	3.90	3.67	3.50	3.36	3.26	3.17	3.03	2.89	2.74	2.66	2.58	2.49	2.40	2.31	2.21
25	7.77	5.57	4.68	4.18	3.85	3.63	3.46	3.32	3.22	3.13	2.99	2.85	2.70	2.62	2.54	2.45	2.36	2.27	2.17
26	7.72	5.53	4.64	4.14	3.82	3.59	3.42	3.29	3.18	3.09	2.96	2.81	2.66	2.58	2.50	2.42	2.33	2.23	2.13
27	7.68	5.49	4.60	4.11	3.78	3.56	3.39	3.26	3.15	3.06	2.93	2.78	2.63	2.55	2.47	2.38	2.29	2.20	2.10
28	7.64	5.45	4.57	4.07	3.75	3.53	3.36	3.23	3.12	3.03	2.90	2.75	2.60	2.52	2.44	2.35	2.26	2.17	2.06
29	7.60	5.42	4.54	4.04	3.73	3.50	3.33	3.20	3.09	3.00	2.87	2.73	2.57	2.49	2.41	2.30	2.23	2.14	2.03
30	7.56	5.39	4.51	4.02	3.70	3.47	3.30	3.17	3.07	2.98	2.84	2.70	2.55	2.47	2.39	2.30	2.21	2.11	2.01
40	7.31	5.18	4.31	3.83	3.51	3.29	3.12	2.99	2.89	2.80	2.66	2.52	2.37	2.29	2.20	2.11	2.02	1.92	1.80
60	7.08	4.98	4.13	3.65	3.34	3.12	2.95	2.82	2.72	2.63	2.50	2.35	2.20	2.12	2.03	1.94	1.84	1.73	1.60
120	6.85	4.79	3.95	3.48	3.17	2.96	2.79	2.66	2.56	2.47	2.34	2.19	2.03	1.95	1.86	1.76	1.66	1.53	1.38
8	6.63	4.61	3.78	3.32	3.02	2.80	2.64	2.51	2.41	2.32	2.18	2.04	1.88	1.79	1.70	1.59	1.47	1.32	1.00

[a]Adapted with permission from *Biometrika Tables for Statisticians*, 2nd ed., Vol. 1, Pearson, E. S. and Hartly, H. O., Eds., Cambridge University Press, New York, 1958.
[b]n_1 = degrees of freedom for numerator.

(b) Analysis of Variance Table and F-Ratios

Source of Variation	Degrees of Freedom	Sum of Squares	Mean Square	F-Ratio	Significance (p-values)
Samples	4	95.3	23.8	136	≦0.01
Judges	2	0.217	0.108	0.6	
Interaction	8	1.20	0.150	0.9	
Residual error	15	2.625	0.175		
Total	29	99.34			

The degrees of freedom in the preceding table are one minus the number of samples and one minus the number of judges for the main effects. The interaction degrees of freedom is obtained by multiplying the two main effect degrees of freedom. The total degrees of freedom is one minus the total number of observations; one degree of freedom rests with the overall average and 15 are left for the residual error term. The sums of squares are sums of the squared deviations of the individual values from the appropriate mean and the mean squares are the sum of squares divided by their degrees of freedom. The F-ratio compares each mean square to the residual mean square of 0.175. For example, the critical F-value for samples with 4 and 15 degrees of freedom is 4.89 at the 1% risk level (Table 6c). The calculated value of 136 (23.8 ÷ 0.175) exceeds this by far. Thus, two or more sample means are statistically different.

H. Multiple Comparisons

1. Least Significant Difference (LSD)

If the F-ratio in an analysis of variance table shows the treatments or samples to be significant, then the least significant difference between means is of interest. Two means are statistically different if they differ by an amount as large as the LSD. Many analysis of variance programs include the LSD values. They can be calculated as follows

$$\text{LSD} = t \cdot \sqrt{\frac{2 \cdot \text{EMS}}{n}}$$

where EMS is the residual error mean square, t is the student's t-value with the degrees of freedom equal to that for the residual mean square (15 in the example in G. Analysis of Variance, Section 3 (b) G3(b)) at a certain alpha risk, usually 0.05, and n is the number of observations contained in each sample average.

The LSD for samples in the example in G3(*b*) is

$$2.13 \cdot \sqrt{\frac{2 \cdot 0.175}{6}} = 0.5$$

The LSD for judges in G3(*b*) is

$$2.13 \cdot \sqrt{\frac{2 \cdot 0.175}{10}} = 0.4$$

It is helpful to plot the sample averages

$$\pm \frac{1}{2} \cdot \text{LSD}$$

to display the differences graphically as shown in Fig. 1. Samples with LSD intervals that do not overlap are statistically different. Note that the significant ordering of these samples from low to high is 3; 1 and 2; 4 and 5. The judge averages could also be plotted.

2. Other Tests for Multiple Comparisons

There are other tests that can be used to compare several means such as the Duncan Multiple Range Test and the Dunnett Test. These are less commonly used and are not detailed here (see Steele and Torrie, 1960).

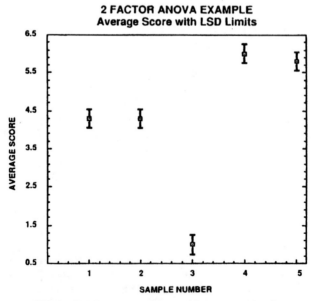

FIG. 1—*Sample averages showing differences graphically.*

I. Threshold Determination

(*a*) Determining an absolute or a difference threshold for a group of people is a two-step process. First, a series of trials is performed to determine each individual's threshold. Then, given a set of individual thresholds, a group threshold is calculated using an agreed upon measure of central tendency (for example, geometric mean, arithmetic mean, median, etc.).

(*b*) For each individual, a series of concentrations of the stimulus are presented on each of several occasions (that is, test sessions). If necessary, the concentrations are adjusted from session to session to ensure that the individual's threshold is contained well within the range tested.

(*c*) For each evaluation a judgment is made as to whether the stimulus was noticed. Typically, forced-choice methods are used (for example, triangle, duo-trio, 3-AFC (that is, 3-alternative forced choice), etc.). A test session consists of a set of forced-choice tests; one for each concentration of stimulus tested. At each concentration, a test sample is evaluated with a reference sample. For absolute thresholds, the reference sample contains none of the stimulus, while for difference thresholds the reference sample contains a fixed, perceivable concentration of the stimulus.

(*d*) The results of the evaluations are used to estimate the proportion of the time the individual detected the stimulus at each concentration. The observed proportion of correct selections is adjusted for the expected proportion of correct guesses, depending on the test method employed. For example, in a triangle test or a 3-AFC test one would expect approximately 1/3 correct selections by chance alone. Therefore, the observed proportion is adjusted using

$$P_a = \frac{3P_o - 1}{2}$$

where

P_o = observed proportion of correct selections and
P_a = adjusted proportion.

(For a duo-trio test the adjustment is $P_a = 2P_o - 1$.)

(*e*) Example of one individual's responses from ten test sessions using a 3-AFC procedure. (A "1" denotes a correct selection of the test sample; a "0" denotes an incorrect selection.)

Concentration 1 was correctly selected in only three of the ten trials, while concentration 4 was correctly selected 8 out of 10 times.

Session	Stimulus Concentration			
	1	2	3	4
1	0	0	1	1
2	0	1	0	1
3	1	1	1	1
4	0	0	0	1
5	0	1	1	0
6	1	0	0	1
7	0	0	0	0
8	0	1	1	1
9	1	0	1	1
10	0	0	1	1
Observed frequency	3	4	6	8
Observed proportion	0.3	0.4	0.6	0.8
Adjusted proportion	0.0	0.1	0.4	0.7

(*f*) Procedure

1. For each individual, tally the adjusted proportion of times each concentration of the stimulus was noticed. This is shown in the last row of the table.

2. Construct a graph with the adjusted proportions on the *y*-axis and the concentration values (or their logarithms) on the *x*-axis. Plot the adjusted proportions versus concentration and draw a smooth curve through the points.

3. Note where the line crosses the 0.50 point on the *y*-axis and, at that point, drop a straight line from the curve to the *x*-axis. The point on the *x*-axis denotes the concentration of the stimulus which is that individual's threshold (for example, approximately 3.33 in this example).

(*g*) If the concentration of the stimulus in the reference sample is zero, then the threshold determined in Step *f* is an absolute threshold. If the concentration of the stimulus in the reference sample is greater than zero, then the threshold determined in Step *f* is a difference threshold.

(*h*) The group threshold, absolute or difference, is calculated by locating the "center" of the group of individuals' thresholds. This is done by calculating an agreed upon measure of central tendency, such as the geometric mean, the arithmetic mean, or the median.

Bibliography

ASTM E18, *Sensory Evaluation of the Appearance of Materials, STP 545,* American Society for Testing and Materials, Philadelphia, 1973.

ASTM, E 679-91, *Determination of Odor and Taste Thresholds by a Forced-Choice Ascending Concentration Series of Limits,* ASTM Standards Volume 15.07, American Society for Testing and Materials, Philadelphia, 1991.

ASTM, E 1432-91, *Defining and Calculating Individual and Group Sensory Thresholds from Forced-Choice Data Sets of Intermediate Size,* ASTM Standards Volume 15.07, American Society for Testing and Materials, Philadelphia, 1991.

ASTM MNL 7, *Manual on Presentation of Data and Control Chart Analysis, 6th edition,* American Society for Testing and Materials, Philadelphia, 1990.

Dixon, W. J. and Massey, F. J., Jr., *Introduction to Statistical Analysis,* McGraw-Hill, New York, 1969.

Gacula, M. C. and Singh, J., *Statistical Methods in Food and Consumer Research,* Academic Press, Orlando, FL, 1984.

Grant, E. I. and Leavenworth, R. S., *Statistical Quality Control,* McGraw-Hill, New York, 1972.

Hochberg, Y. and Tamhane, A. C., *Multiple Comparison Procedures,* John Wiley and Sons, New York, 1987.

Hunter, W. G. and Hunter, J. S., *Statistics for Experimenters, G.E.P. Box,* John Wiley and Sons, New York, 1978.

Meilgaard, M., Civile, G. V., and Carr, B. T., *Sensory Evaluation Techniques,* 2nd edition, CRC Press, Inc., Boca Raton, FL, 1991.

Siegal, S., *Nonparametric Statistics for the Behavioral Science,* McGraw-Hill, New York, 1956.

Steele, R. G. D. and Torrie, J. H., *Principles and Procedures of Statistics,* McGraw-Hill, New York, 1960.

Index

A

Affective testing, 8–10, 73–77
  hedonic scale method, 73–75
  orientation and training of
    respondents, 11
  paired preference test, 75–77
Alternative hypothesis, 83
Analysis of variance, 102–107
Analytical tests
  orientation and training of
    respondents, 10–11
  respondents, 5–8
A-not-A test, 29–30

B

Bias, sources of, 21–23
Bipolar scales, 43–44

C

Characterization of difference, 35–36
Chi-square test, 98–102
Codes, for samples, 14
Comfort, testing room, 5
Complex sorting tasks, 34–35
Critical values, power tables, 88–93
Cues, 14

D

Degree of difference, 35
Descriptive analysis, 58–70
  flavor profile method, 58–62
  general rating scale for attribute
    intensity, 67–69
  Quantitative Descriptive Analysis
    (QDA), 63–65
  Spectrum Descriptive Analysis, 65–67
  texture profile method, 62–63

  time-intensity method, 69–70
Dilution techniques, 56–57
Duo-trio test, 26–27
  significance of results, 86, 88
  statistical procedures, 84–86

E

End anchors, scales, 43
Experimenter, attitudes, 14–15

F

Flavor profile method, 58–62
Forced choice discrimination tests, 25–36
  A-not-A test, 29–30
  characterization of difference, 35–36
  complex sorting tasks, 34–35
  degree of difference, 35
  design, 32–33
  duo-trio test, 26–27
  interpretation of results, 35
  method selection, 34
  multiple standards test, 30–32
  paired difference test, 28–29
  sample size, 34
  3-alternative forced choice, 27–28
  triangle (triangular) test, 6, 25–26
F-ratio, 104–107

G

Generalized t-test, 93–94
General rating scale for attribute
  intensity, 67–69
Graphic scale, 40

113

H

Hedonic scale method, 73–75
Humidity control, sample presentation, 18
Hypothesis testing, 82–86

J

Just-about-right scaling method, 50–52

L

Laboratory
   layout, 3–4
   location, 3
Least significant difference, 107–108
Length of scale formats, 42–43
Lighting, laboratory, 4–5
Location, testing laboratory, 3

M

Magnitude estimation, 45–46
Method of constant stimuli, 56
Method of limits, 56
Motivation, of respondents, 11–12
Multiple comparisons, 107–108
Multiple standards test, 30–32
Multiple tests of significance, 87

N

Null hypothesis, 83
Numerical scale, 41

O

Odor control, laboratory, 4
One-sided alternative hypothesis, 83
One-sided paired comparison,
   significance of results, 86, 88

P

Paired-comparison results, two-tailed, 85, 88
Paired difference test, 28–29
Paired preference test, 75–77
Paired t-test, 94–95
Panel size, 7–8

Panel training (see Respondents, orientation and training)
Physical conditions, of testing, 3–5
Physiological factors, influencing sensory verdicts, 21–23
Physiological sensitivity, of respondents, 12–13
Pictorial scales, 42
Power, triangle tests, 88–93
Preference test, 36, 75–77
Probability, 83–84
Proportions, t-test, 95–96
Psychological control, of respondents, 13–15

Q

Quantitative Descriptive Analysis (QDA), 63–65

R

Rank order, 46–47
   data analysis, 48
Rating scales, 39–45
   applications, 39
   end anchors for scales, 43
   graphic scale, 40
   length of scale formats, 42–43
   numerical scale, 41
   pictorial scales, 42
   scale of standards, 41–42
   unipolar and bipolar scales, 43–44
   verbal scale, 41
Reliability of results, 87
Respondents, 5–15
   affective tests, 8–10
   analytical tests, 5–8
   motivation, 11–12
   orientation and training, 10–11, 58
   physiological sensitivity, 12–13
   psychological control, 13–15
   screening, 5–6

S

Samples
   amount of, 18
   codes, 14

elimination of appearance and other
 factors, 18-19
number of, 19-20
order of presentation, 19
preparation, 16-17, 55
presentation, 17-24
selection, 16
size, forced choice discrimination
 tests, 34
temperature/humidity control, 18
Scale of standards, 41-42
Scaling, 38-52
 data divisions, 38-39
 just-about-right scaling method, 50-52
 magnitude estimation, 45-46
 rank order, 46-47
 rating scales, 39-45
Screening, respondents, 5-6
Sorting tasks, complex, 34-35
Spectrum Descriptive Analysis, 65-67
Statistical errors, 83-84
Statistical procedures, 79-110
 analysis of variance, 102-107
 chi-square test, 98-102
 critical values and power tables, 88-93
 hypothesis testing, 82-86
 least significant difference, 107-108
 limitations and qualifications, 87
 multiple comparisons, 107-108
 reference to prepared tables, 87-93
 significance, 79, 87
  paired-comparison results in two-
   tailed, 85, 88

results in duo-trio or one-sided
 paired comparison, 86, 88
theoretical basis, 87
threshold determination, 109-110
t-test, 93-98
Statistical significance, 84-86
Statistical terms, definitions, 79-82
Symbols, 81

T

Temperature control, sample
 presentation, 18
Texture profile method, 62-63
3-alternative forced choice, 27-28
Threshold determination, 109-110
Threshold methods, 54-57
 dilution techniques, 56-57
 method of constant stimuli, 56
 method of limits, 56
 sample preparation, 55
Time-intensity method, 69-70
Training and orientation of respondents,
 10-11, 58
Triangle (triangular) test, 6, 25-26
t-test, 93-98
 average against fixed value, 97-98
Two-sided alternative hypothesis, 83

U

Unipolar scales, 43-44

V

Verbal scale, 41